The Best is Yet to Come

The Best is Yet to Come

AMANDA HANCOCK
Foreword by Jamie Like and Anita Frazer
Introduction by Dan Hancock

© 2017 Amanda Hancock
All rights reserved.

ISBN-13: 9781975802448
ISBN-10: 1975802446
Library of Congress Control Number: 2017913566
CreateSpace Independent Publishing Platform
North Charleston, South Carolina

Foreword

By Jamie Like and Anita Frazer

The first time we met Dan and Amanda, they came into our winery tasting room, and almost instantly, we knew that we liked them. As a small business owner, you sometimes get a feel for people as they walk through your doors. On this particular day, we saw a young, newly married couple, both equally intelligent, funny, and kind. Amanda shared that she was a social worker, and Dan told us that he was in the process of opening a law practice in Evansville. After tasting all of our wines, they decided upon a bottle and went out on our patio to enjoy it, along with the beauty of the day.

After a half hour or so, Dan came into the tasting room to pick out some cheese and crackers for him and Amanda, and he chatted with us for several minutes while he was there. Amanda ended up coming in to look for him, and we all got to chatting together once again. That ended up being the first of many of their visits to see us at Ruby Moon over a period of about eight years.

About a year after we first met Dan and Amanda, Amanda told us that she was going to culinary school and that she had always loved to cook. A few visits later, Amanda told us she was no longer working as a social worker and that she was working for a small upscale deli and grocery in Newburgh called Vecchio's.

We stopped in to see Amanda at Vecchio's from time to time, and eventually she told us that she and Dan were going to buy Vecchio's and that she would run it as the head chef. That was the start of our love affair with Vecchio's—its amazing food, great staff, and awesome wine and craft beer selection. We asked Amanda to come to Ruby Moon at one point and teach a class on cheese making; it was well attended. We loved collaborating with Amanda and Dan and shared a very genuine and caring friendship with them. Probably six years ago, we started a tradition of playing golf on May 22, for both Dan's and Anita's birthdays. We had such great fun and usually laughed nonstop the whole day.

A couple of years ago, we stopped in Vecchio's one Sunday for lunch, and one of their staff members, Jessica, told us that Amanda was sick and that Dan had taken her to an urgent-care center to find out what was wrong with her. That was the beginning of what would become a very long, painful nightmare for them both. Over a period of a few months, we saw Amanda go from being a strong, confident, celebrated chef to a sickly, weak, jaundiced young woman who was becoming a shell of who she used to be. After a lengthy period of jumping through numerous hoops and being on a waiting list for a liver transplant, they finally got the call. Dan and Amanda headed to Indy, and it seemed, for a moment, that the wheels were turning around and that Amanda would soon be on the road to recovery.

Shortly after the surgery, however, things went terribly wrong when Amanda slipped into a coma, in which she stayed for a period of several weeks. When she finally came out of the coma, it was apparent that a lot of damage had been done and that she would have to not only regain the abilities to eat, walk, and speak, but that she would also be profoundly changed forever. It was during the time when Amanda was sick, awaiting the liver transplant, and the several months she spent trying to come back to some semblance of herself afterward, that we were witness to the greatest love story we have ever seen.

To say that Dan was selfless during the time that Amanda was sick and recovering doesn't begin to describe the man we saw Dan become. We watched Dan and saw a superhuman being whose strength, both physically and emotionally, was endless. We remarked a couple of times during those grueling months that their story would make one heck of a book, and that is what has brought us here to the point.

So it is with much joy, love, and honor that we have written the foreword for this amazing book. Watching Amanda's determination during her long, slow, painful, and frustrating recovery was nothing short of watching a miracle unfold over time. If we can ever become half the people that Dan and Amanda are, we will consider ourselves to be doing quite well. We love you both immensely!

Jamie and Anita

Introduction

By Dan Hancock

There are some stories that must be told. This is one of those stories. It embodies the meaning of "Till death do us part." This isn't my story, but I'm immersed in it. The smartest person I know entrusted me with *the* decision. She told me what to do, and I never doubted her, even under the unbearable pressure, enduring things that no one will ever know. I am proud to say I am holding "a handful of spades," and my girl is proof that nothing is impossible. She casts a very long shadow; I'm just honored to carry the water.

—Dan, "The Water Boy"

This was the original intro I wrote; then, I was told to make it better. That's a big task compared to what you are about to read. No one will ever know everything except me. Except me.

I hope this is good enough, Amanda.

—Big D

ix

One

Of course the first chapter has to be all about *me*. Before I got a liver transplant, I had been diagnosed with kidney disease. This led to hours of hours of dialysis, which means four hours of being hooked up to a machine with nothing to do but look at other sick people. I tried to pursue different hobbies, such teaching myself to knit with the help of my mom (her name is Daphine; most of my friends call her Momma D). I also gained a rich appreciation for good music.

In 2014 I was diagnosed with liver disease. What causes that? I was quite overweight, and I enjoyed adult drinks too much (boo!). So I was put on the waiting list. I was put on the list on January 7 of that year, and I was the first on the list because of the score of my MELD, which stands for Model for End-Stage Liver Disease. My score was so high that they were afraid that I could die. They told Dan that it could take a while for me to get on a liver-disease list.

I got ahead of myself. I could tell about all the tests; I had to go through many tests, such as a Pap smear, a mammogram, a stress test, a weight test, a dental exam, a respiratory test, and a kidney exam.

I got put on the list on January 7. This was a very emotional call for me because I was excited and scared all at the same time. Dan has a picture of me listening in on the phone. I looked so sick and orange. I was orange because of the buildup of bilirubin, which is processed in the liver. If there are problems with your liver, it will cause jaundice, which causes your skin to turn bright yellow and your eyes bright orange. Yes, you will look like a monster. Guess what? You just have to suck it up, buttercup. I know that sounds harsh, but it's an unforgiving disease.

We finally got *the* call that there was a liver ready just for *me*! We only had three hours to get there. Luckily we had a bag packed, so we hopped into the SUV and were on our way! I can't express this enough: don't put yourself in this position. Avoid this at all costs. It's terrible, so do me a favor: please take good care of yourself.

I forgot to mention that I also got diagnosed with something that most people call ODS, which stands for osmotic demyelination syndrome. Say that over and over three times as fast as you can (heh heh). You are welcome!

So I got my transplant on January 11. It took four hours, but I had some trouble waking up (they gave me some really good medications). So when I did wake up, I saw Dan standing over me with love and worry. But he was in tears of joy. I was in tears of pain. He said that everything went well, and our families were all there and couldn't wait to see me.

I came out with a ventilator, but it came out soon enough, and I went on regular oxygen. It was hard to talk; I was so anxious to see everyone and stressed my voice too much, so Dan sent everyone out so we could have time to be alone with each other. I had never been so happy. It went on for days, and I loved him so much. I was, and am still, in love with him. On the third day, I asked him to go back to his hotel because he was asking too many questions. I know he was

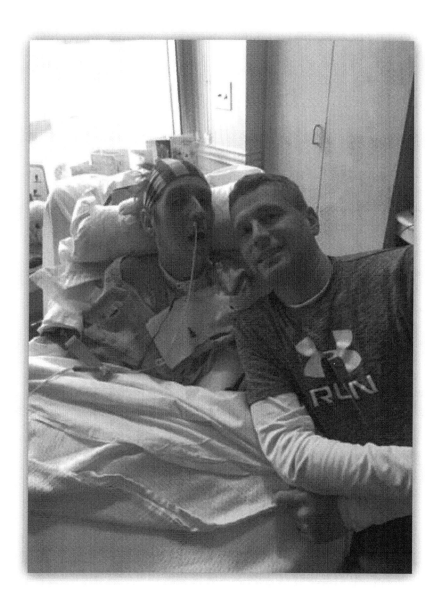

worried about me and was so relieved, but I just needed some rest. So I gave him a kiss, told him I loved him, and said I couldn't wait to see him in the morning. Those were the last words I said to him for two weeks. I slipped into a coma.

Apparently I had two seizures during that time. They had to trach me because I couldn't breathe on my own. People were starting to worry that I wouldn't make it through. But, ta-da! I made it through. But I couldn't talk for two months. That's when they sent me to the Rehabilitation Hospital in Indianapolis. I got the best care from the staff. I still work with some of them. I have one fine lady at Saint Mary's in Evansville, Indiana, whom I have nicknamed *the Boss*!

Now it's time to talk about physical therapy. I have been lucky to have a few good physical therapists. They have taught me several different ways to exercise. The first physical therapist I can remember was very nice (but short), but he is the one who helped get out of my wheelchair. He got me walking on parallel bars. Then, he started making games to do on the bars. I had to pick things up off of the bars and put them back. Then I had to walk backward and then on my tiptoes. And then we started tackling stairs. I know that sounds goofy. And trust me, I was very embarrassed because I was a thirty-five-year-old woman having to relearn how to walk. And then I went to a skilled nursing facility, where I met my next physical therapist. There I got to know the gentleman who made me march up and down the hallways with five-pound weights. Talk about tough!

Then I got to go home, and I could go to outpatient physical therapy. That's where I met *the Boss* again! At first I couldn't remember her from when I was in the hospital, but as soon as she started my workout program, it all came right back to me.

I quickly learned that she wasn't willing to let me slack. Trust me, I had bad words going through my head several times, but she and Dan gradually built my confidence in myself. Then I got to graduate

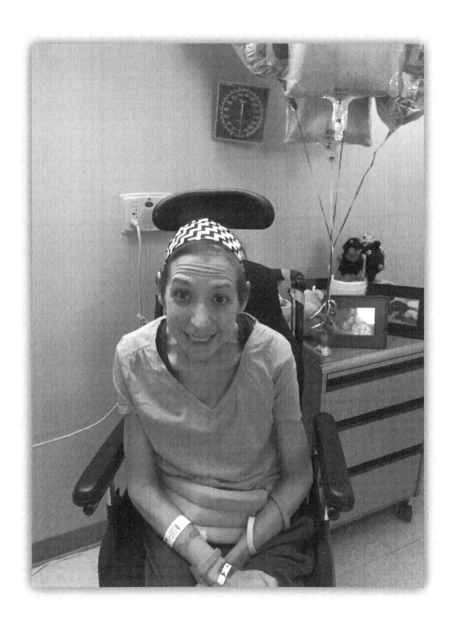

to the trapeze-looking thing. I was really scared when I saw it, but she explained that it was there to support me as my tasks began to advance. So then I was able to work up to walking on the treadmill for ten minutes with only one hand on the mill. It took quite a while to work up to that, but it was so satisfying when I could. Then I starting walking backward, walking on foam, riding a bike, doing sit-and-stands, and keeping my balance on a board that rocked back and forth. And then she started timing each of my tests, which was required so she could show progress to my insurance. It's part of having personal insurance. So that meant I had to walk one thousand feet in six minutes. And there were also obstacle courses that entailed walking up and down steps, stepping over cones, and lying down on a mat and getting back up on my own. That's harder than one would think. We do it every day, right? We are never timed to do it. You know that at the end of the day, you will be tired and sore, but when you get you get up the next day, you will feel great, and you will be proud of your accomplishments that day. Trust me, I have gone to bed feeling like my hind end has fallen off, but I'm always happy to find out that's still there! I will always tell people it is the best choice to recover, period!

Even yesterday, March 17, 2016, she had me walking up and down a hill (on grass, mind you), and then she started throwing a ball at me. I felt like it was torture, but she kept telling me that I would feel great this morning. Guess what? I felt terrible this morning. I know I can type it now, because I know she won't read this for a few weeks. So I should be safe, right? And then yesterday, she had me stand on a minitrampoline, and she held onto me while she had Dan throw a ball at me. It sounds like torture, and it felt like it yesterday—and again today. No pain, no gain, right?

Another outlet is to find local programs, maybe at a local university, college, or local YMCA. I'm sure they all will be welcoming and excited to help. Just know that it is an ongoing process. It is well worth it.

Then I was going to start occupational therapy. A study found evidence that, in fact, makes a case for occupational therapy post–liver transplant. It says that people benefit from programs that can make key improvements to maximize self-satisfaction. Who doesn't need that? I know that I do.

I realized a few days ago that it was officially Kidney Disease Day! So Dan and I always choose to wear a bright-orange shirts. Orange is the color that supports people with kidney disease. I've had it, and we both have family members who have suffered from it. It's very hard to deal with it; some people can just fix it with dialysis, which I've already discussed, but some folks need full transplants. That is why our families both support Donate Life. We have bracelets that are green, which is the color that has been chosen to represent the cause. You can probably find them online.

OK, on to my occupational therapist friends, both from Woodlands in Newburgh, Indiana, and from Saint Mary's in Evansville, Indiana. They have been very patient with me. They know I hate the eye patch, but my therapist insisted that I wear it every session. She even wants me to wear it at home (yeah, right). But I have to admit that it does work.

Then there were my very patient speech therapists. They were the folks who helped me remember how to speak again and eat again. I know it sounds funny, but I had practically stopped eating shortly after my liver transplant. I had just lost my appetite, so they had to put feeding tube into my stomach. It lived in my stomach for eight long months. When it came out, I had trouble acclimating to food again, which frustrated me because I had gone back to school and become a professional chef. I even owned a local Italian restaurant. I had developed a good palate. Now I couldn't even stand eating anything. So they had to start me on Jell-O. Seriously? I was offended, but anything harder choked me up. Then it was crackers, and then it was bread. Then I started getting salt and pepper, and soup. And then

I got to eat lunch meat sandwiches. I know this is boring to read, but we all have had family members who have lost their abilities to swallow. So please be patient with these folks. You will notice how much they will appreciate you for being patient with them.

OK, I am always concerned about food. But I need to discuss how they helped me speak more loudly—although if anyone knows me, I'm not a quiet person. I am one of those people who was born without a filter between my mouth and my mind. But somewhere along the way, I lost my volume. So the occupational therapists had the task of helping me find my voice again. It took countless times of me having to say "Ahhh" over and over until I could say it loudly enough that everyone could hear me. Apparently some people don't like it when I use it on them. Back to that lack of a filter, it always bites me in the rear. I had to get Botox three times twice, once in late April 2014, in the back of my neck. This allowed me to hold my head up on my own. Apparently I didn't appreciate it, because I had no say in it. I now realize that there was no way that I could have understood that at this particular time. And the second time I had Botox shots, I got two shots in September, one in my pectoral muscle, and then two in my elbow. One was above my elbow, and one was below my elbow. I still shake from my ODS.

I would like to talk about the effects of my struggles. I needed a lot of support to get better. This included support from members of my family and from Dan's family as well. Also we had a *ton* of friends who raised money through fund-raisers, like pancake dinners, selling yellow bracelets, and a spaghetti dinner, and they collected aluminum cans. Dan and I were so grateful for all their help. We can never thank them enough.

I would like to talk about the effects on our families, friends, and, most importantly, my husband, Dan. He spent many days sleeping on chairs and in hotel rooms. Mind you, I was in a hospital, rehab center,

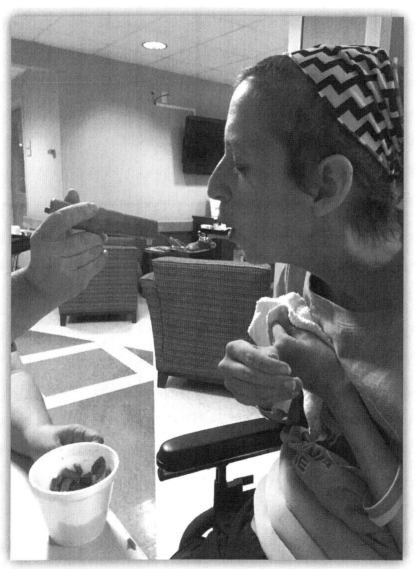

Me being fed because I had no use of my arms yet.

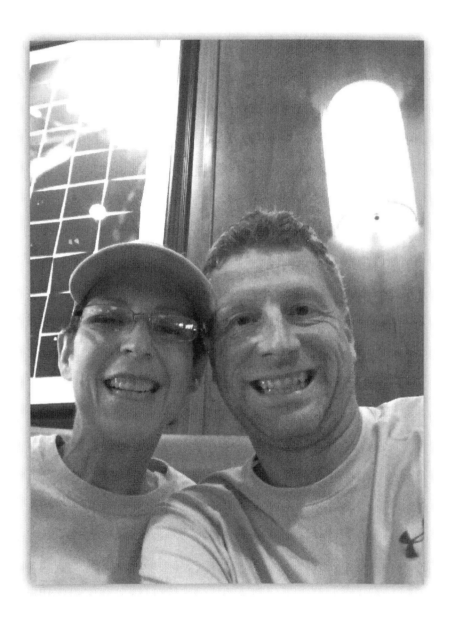

or nursing facility for eight long months of 2015. That's a long time for anyone to wait for someone to wake up, learn to walk and talk, and eat and breathe on her own again at thirty-five years old. Dan was there every step of the way, sleeping in a chair next to me. Sometimes the nurses would put me in a room with a couch so he could stay with me. Some days he would go to a hotel room so he could actually sleep. He has earned over three months in the hotel rooms.

I would like to talk about our families. I'll start with mine. My family is fairly small; there is me (obviously). My dad is named Jim. And then there is my mom, Daphine, otherwise known as Momma D. I have one sister, Debby (don't dare to spell it wrong). She is the best auditor in the area. Then there is my supersmart niece. I have always considered myself smart, but Emily can outthink me every day. I have secretly always been jealous. (I guess it's no secret now.) We used to sit down and work out word searches together, but I got tired of having to concede because she always won. Here is a funny story about one time when we were getting dressed to start pictures. Emily won't like that I'm telling this, but oh, well; it's my book. As she was putting on her dress, a seam busted. Immediately she panicked. But luckily Mary, Dan's cousin's wife, jumped in and was able to sew it up. Emergency diverted!

Then there is John; he is the brother I always wanted to have. Every time I decided to pack up and move, whether it was across the street or to a different state, he was right there to help me out.

Dan and I got married on August 7, 2004. It was an evening wedding in a candlelit gazebo. It was everything I wanted and then some. Right as John and I were turning to walk down the aisle, he leaned over to me and asked, "Are you sure you're ready for this?" It caught me off guard, but when we turned to walk, I saw Dan, and I knew that he was the one for me.

We went to the receiving line while everyone went back into the gazebo and set it up for the reception. It was mostly done by my sister and the rest of *our* new extended family. There was so much food that it was hard to get it all in.

And we get to Big D's family. Bear with me; it is a huge family. His mom and dad have become my family, too. His mom is named Janice (she made me put in here that she is a fabulous genius). She is a great seamstress; she can embroider. Dad's name is Frank, and he is fantastic with woodworking. He has one brother, Jason, and a sister-in-law, Sarah, and they have a baby named Amelia. Dan had five grandparents. In total there are twenty-two aunts and uncles and twenty-six first cousins. I told you it was a big family. And now I had to meet everyone and try to remember their names.

So we finally got through the crowd so we could get to Nashville, Tennessee. We had to change clothes and get on the road because were catching a plane to Mexico the next morning. We were both hungry, because you don't get to eat at your own reception, as you are busy glad-handing and saying your thank-yous. We stopped and got some food. He drove while I opened the gift cards to see how much cash we got as gifts. Everyone does that, right? Well, that's what everyone told me. So we were well on our way to our hotel, which should be exciting, right? I had many nerves and thoughts of "This it, and what should I expect?" Well, that's not how it went at all. We were so tired. It took a few hours to get the bobby pins out of my hair. Then we settled into bed for "you know," but I was caught off guard when my loving new husband decided to be romantic. *Ooh la la*, he started kissing me, and he moved his hand, and then *crash*! He fell right off of the bed. One would think I should be concerned, but no. I just rolled over and busted out laughing. What kind of wife was I going to be? I guess I've done OK; it's been twelve years this year. Well, we haven't gotten off the honeymoon yet.

We arrived at our hotel in the Mayan Riviera. It was stunning; it had pool that played music under the water. It sounds odd, but if you were on a float, you could dunk your head under the water and hear the music. There was also a labyrinth, where one could spend hours walking and trying to figure it out. We had a beautiful room. It had a full minibar, all for free! It also had sunroof right over our hot tub. It was everything we wanted. We met our personal butler; he was awesome. So he took us down to the hotel bar. He gave us his card in case we got lost. Was it a bad thing to get lost in paradise? He ordered us unlimited margaritas. Well, they brought us chips and spicy cheese dip. And we were professionals at drinking margaritas. We didn't realize exactly what Mexican margaritas were. Apparently they are *all* tequila and a bit of lime. We both lost track of how many we had. Remember the personal butler we had? We had to call him to get back to our room. Little did we know they also put a nice champagne in our room. You can't let that go to waste, right? So we had to drink that, too. We happened to have to need to go to an in-service the next morning. Guess who spent all night in the shower tossing up *her* cookies? Needless to say, Dan went alone. He said he was not the only single guy down there. I spent that time in the hot tub with a bottle of water.

I got a "great" surprise when Big D came back. He had talked to the guys downstairs. They convinced him he needed to climb the stairs at Chichen Itza. Obviously, I wasn't feeling it. It was hot and sticky. I hadn't thought we were going to leave the hotel, so I had only packed a swimsuit, a tank top, and some pajama pants. So Dan started up the mountain, and I sat on a tree stump at the base of the pyramid, drinking water. The tour was amazing. I didn't realize the advanced technology that this culture had in that period of time. The ride back was a culture shock to me, too. They handed out free beer. I knew that wasn't legal, but Dan reminded me that we were in Mexico. Oh yeah, I knew that, right?

So we got to spend the rest of our honeymoon sitting out on our balcony and experiencing *real* Mexican food. We tried figuring out the labyrinth. We (I mean I) went to the spa. We spent time on the beach. But, of course, it couldn't end on a good note. I got stung by a bee. My neck began to swell, which freaked me out. It was during the time when there were stories about the weird diseases found in countries abroad. So we went running down to the resort pharmacy to see if we could find some allergy medicine. All we could find was medicine that was labeled with a brand that we knew. I took it, and we were off to the airport to come home. Dan ate a piece of pizza from a place that we have in the States. I didn't eat, as I was doped up on allergy drugs.

About the time that we landed in Memphis, got through customs, and got our bags, Dan got me seated in a chair. He had to "go." It was important at that point. We then got swept onto a plane to Nashville to get back to our car. It was a memorable time.

We spent the next few years traveling. We went to Chicago, Las Vegas, San Francisco, and Napa. And we stayed with our good friends at Ruby Moon Winery in Henderson, Kentucky. Our all-time favorite was West Baden Springs in French Lick, Indiana. We also went to 21c Museum Hotel in Louisville, Kentucky; they have wonderful art exhibits, many of which are local. If you ever find someone who stays there, ask them about the men's restrooms—they're pretty funny. We were close to the Louisville Slugger museum, and the Muhammad Ali Center is close to it, too. There are a ton of eclectic art exhibits and restaurants all over town. And my some of my most favorite memories come from the famous Churchill Downs.

Dan and I have been to the derby twice. One time we were able to take my family. It is so fun because you get to go and buy new duds. The ladies get new dresses and *fancy* hats. The gentlemen get nice suits. Dan always gets out his seersucker suit and his favorite suspenders and bow ties (which he always wears). The second time we went with my work family, Frank and his wife, Gina, and our good friends, our then–pastry chef and her husband. We all got along like a family, and we had the best of times. Frank gave us all the courage to walk around the surrounding neighborhoods and experience their homemade foods.

Dan and I also went to Lexington, Kentucky, where we got to watch the *CATS*. I was even able to fight my way down to the floor to get the famous three. True fans will know what that means. We went to the horse park to see some of the most famous thoroughbreds, and we got see a show with all of the breeds.

I've had a wonderful life, but I did not realize how much I could possibly learn about my diseases. I have always been a good student, and I enjoy learning. But this time I took the hard way to learn my lesson. I hope this inspires you to study up and take a better road than I chose to.

Liver disease is too complicated to explain in a few words, so bear with me. I thought it wasn't me causing it. That's what I tried to tell myself, but that was a lie. I suffered from fatty liver disease, being overweight, an overuse of alcoholic beverages, and poor eating habits. That seemed to be the imperfect solution for my issues. Like I said previously, it is a long, painful, drawn-out process. If you find yourself in this position, you must be physically and mentally prepared. It important to go to all the classes the hospital offers. You may think that you have done all the research you possibly could do. You haven't. There are antirejection drugs that will have to be taken *every* day of your life. You cannot live without these drugs. People do not realize how incredibly important this is. One can never prepare oneself for this entire process without professional help.

It is a good time to surround yourself with family and trusted friends. Find a good therapist to vent to. It too much for one person to take on him- or herself. There is too much anxiety about what could go wrong. How long does it take to get better? It is time to get back to the things you loved to do. If not, you will start to get depressed and sad, and then you will start feeling bad for yourself. Worst thing *ever*—that's exactly what I did, and now I have to take a handful of medications and get physical, occupational, and speech therapy twice a week.

I have found a couple of studies regarding liver transplants and the recovery process. If you get a transplant manual, read it over and over; it could be a lifesaver—literally. It spells out the recommended diet and appropriate exercises posttransplant. It explains exactly how much water one needs to drink. When you see the cup, you will think, *There is no way that can fit in me.* Guess what? You have to drink that cup three times a day. Good luck to you!

Studies have shown that nearly 10 percent of patients do not survive the first three months. That was enough to scare me. Furthermore, "In several cases the QOL scores stayed low as these individuals were unprepared for the potential complications associated with this difficult surgery."[1] This perfectly described me. By the way, QOL means quality of life.

That is important to think about when you are battling this disease, especially if you are anything like me. I spent all of my time feeling guilty that someone had to lose his or her life so I could live after I had abused my own body.

---

1 Scott, Winslow, Krause, and Bah, *Impact of Medical, Health Related, Social, and Occupational Factors on Post-Liver Transplant Recovery: A Longitudinal Study* (Place: Publisher, Year), page number.

Two

It's time to learn to cook the diet that was given to you. There are certain things you can and can't eat. So here is a guide to the dos and don'ts of eating the ways your doctor said you should. We will start with the good list.

- Go low sodium, and with that, you must drink a lot of water. You can put low-calorie drink mixes in it. Or you can drink tea with only sweetener, no sugar. I almost forgot my personal favorite—coffee. I like it black or with some coconut milk in it. Or with two shots of espresso.
- There are low-sugar juices. You can have grape, apple, orange, and any mix of all; my personal favorite is Tang. Who doesn't love Tang? I am afraid that the younger ones don't know what that wonderful invention was; they do not understand how much it meant to us!

- We can't have grapefruit or pomegranate juice, because it affects the way your body absorbs your medications.
- *Do* drink plenty of high-protein drinks, like Boost, Ensure, and Muscle Milk; these will help build muscles. Also drink something called the Green Machine. It looks gross, but it tastes very good. It has green apple, pear, kiwi, mango, bananas, spinach, kale, and wheatgrass.
- Eat a lot of fresh vegetables and fruits. Frozen works, but you get more nutrients from fresh.
- Look for fresh fruits, blueberries, strawberries, raspberries, apples, oranges, grapes, melons, bananas, kiwis…the options are endless.
- If you end up with frozen fruits, add some yogurt and some ice, and just put everything in a blender, and poof! You have a tasty fruit smoothie. Just add some sugar substitute. If you're feeling really creative, add some granola. You will be the best chef in the house.

Now on to some recipes. Remember that we can only use lean meats, such as chicken, turkey, crab, tuna, some salmon, or a small amount of shrimp. You have to be careful because it has a ton of cholesterol. I know that is not a popular fact, but if you have an issue with your liver, you have to look at every aspect of each piece of food that goes into your mouth. Sorry, Charlie, but you have to learn to take care yourself. It stinks, but you will get better faster.

Eat your food groups:

- Protein, such as cheese, milk, eggs, beans, cottage cheese, ice cream, and yogurt.
- Vitamin C, such as lemons, oranges, strawberries, broccoli, cantaloupe, and tomatoes.

- Vitamin A, which includes carrots, sweet potatoes, greens, egg yolks, and liver.
- Zinc, which includes baked potatoes, fruit juices, oatmeal, spinach, and shellfish.
- Iron, which includes peas, liver, sardines, tuna, prune juice, and dried peaches.
- Vitamin E, which includes egg yolks, liver (I am staring to see a pattern here), leafy greens, and whole grains.
- Skin care: it's important—you have to be cleaned frequently; use cream or oil on your hands.

And the most important thing is to drink lots and lots of water. It will keep you hydrated and keep your kidneys working and your bowels moving. If you don't like drinking a whole bottle of water, take sips here and there.

Start simple. Please remember that I am a trained chef, so I may get ahead of myself. First thing, you should go through your spice cabinet and get rid of anything you haven't used in six months. They have probably gone bad by now. Find a good cookbook.

I have my school handbook, which is entitled *Cooking*. It was written by several chefs: Labensky, Hause, and Marel. This is the book that I had in school. It is nearly twelve hundred pages long. Have it all? No way, but I have learned all the basics. Things like the fact that mirepoix is made of two parts onion, one part celery, and one part carrot, all by weight.

Butter = unsalted whole milk; don't substitute skim milk.
TT = to taste.

I have another favorite; it is *The Complete Art of Cooking*, written by Silvie Girard. It starts with how to prepare each product correctly and safely. There are a ton of great recipes, but first I'm going to share some of my own.

Simple Salsa

- 4 large, fresh heirloom tomatoes; score the bottoms with a shallow X, and then put them in a deep pan of hot water. Let them soak until they start to peel themselves. Don't leave them in so long that they cook. Once they are starting to peel, quickly put them in a full ice bath. You will be amazed how easy this makes it.
- A fresh avocado—make sure that it is not bruised, too soft, or too hard.
- 3 cloves of fresh garlic, peeled and run through a press. If you aren't a garlic fan, you can use more or less.
- 1 small batch of green onions; just dice the green parts in small pieces at an angle.
- 1 Tbsp. cumin. If you like it a bit spicy, add some hot sauce or dice up some jalapeño, making sure that you get the seeds and stems out. That is where the spices live.
- 1 handful of fresh cilantro; make sure that it is washed and dried before you chop it up.
- Put the juice of a lime over the salsa, and add in a dash of salt and pepper, to taste.

I forgot the 3 most important things in a kitchen:

- Always wash your hand before you walk into the kitchen and throughout the cooking process, and use hand sanitizer.
- Always wear gloves when touching food that will not be cooked.
- Always have your knives sharpened; if you aren't comfortable doing it, take them to a professional. There; I am done with my speech.

Next stop is my favorite gazpacho.

- 1½ lbs. of vine-ripened tomatoes, peeled, seeded, and chopped
- 1 can of fresh tomato juice
- 1 cucumber, peeled, seeded, and chopped
- ½ chopped onion
- ½ cup chopped red pepper
- 1 small jalapeño, seeded and minced
- ¼ cup olive oil
- 1 garlic clove, minced
- 1 lime, juiced
- 2 tsp. Worcestershire sauce
- ½ tsp. toasted ground cumin
- 1 tsp. kosher salt
- ¼ tsp. freshly ground black pepper
- 2 Tbsp. fresh basil chiffonade (which means to roll them up and cut into small ribbons)
- After peeling the tomatoes, cut out the seeds and pulp, and put them in a strainer to get the juice.
- Chop the tomatoes, and put them in a bowl with the juice. Add the cucumber, garlic, olive oil, lime juice, Worcestershire sauce, cumin, salt, and pepper.
- Put 1½ cup of the soup into a blender, and puree for 15 to 20 seconds.
- Return to the bowl; stir everything together, and let it stand in the fridge and soak for 2 hours.
- When it is time to serve it, serve it with some crackers or some tortilla chips.

Here are some recipes that I came up with some ideas from my favorite cookbooks.

Cold tomato soup

- To serve 4, put 3 cups of tomato juice in the refrigerator to get good and cold.
- Peel a clove of garlic, chop finely, and then grind it on the cutting board with a sturdy knife and some good-quality olive oil.
- Put the tomatoes, juice, garlic, a pinch of sugar, celery salt, and pepper, in serving bowls, and if you like, add some fennel or chervil.

How much do you like artichokes? They get a bad a rep. I think it is just because they look so intimidating to some people. It really is easy. This is a really easy preparation; it takes the artichoke and stuffs it with tomato confit. Don't be discouraged; it's not as hard as it reads.

- Prepare 8 small artichokes by cutting off the woody stems.
- Put the chokes into a steaming basket, and steam them just until tender.
- Then, cut off the outer leaves; cut out the heart and chokes.
- Cut 1 lemon in half, and rub it over the exposed parts of the choke.
- In the meantime, wash 2 tomatoes, and cut them into quarters.
- Chop 2 garlic cloves and onion to taste.
- Stuff the artichokes with the tomato confit, and serve while still warm.

This recipe serves 6 people. Enjoy!

How about green beans with almonds?

- 3½ oz. slivered almonds

- 1 lb. 2 oz. green beans, snapped at the ends and in quarters, washed and dried
- 2–3 fresh white onions, sliced thinly
- 2 Tbsp. olive oil
- 1 bundle of fresh savory (you can usually find it at specialty stores)
- 2–3 Tbsp. crème fraîche; if you can't find it, substitute sour cream.
- Place the slivered almonds in a heavy skillet, and slowly begin to toast them.
- Meanwhile, blanch the green beans in salted and oiled water. Pat the water off them.
- Add the sour cream, the onions, and the warm green beans.
- Toss it all together, and serve on warm plates.
  Serves 4 people.

How about some fall/winter dishes?

<u>Glazed carrots</u>

- You obviously need carrots. Get enough carrots for the number of guests you're having. Either buy baby carrots, or get full-sized carrots. Peel the carrots, and slice them into quarters. Make sure they are washed and dried.
- Honey
- Lime juice
- Garlic powder
- Extra-virgin olive oil
- Sauté the carrots in ¼ cup of olive oil, just until they are bright orange and tender.

- Transfer the hot carrots to a bowl, and toss with the honey, lime juice, garlic powder, and salt and pepper to taste.

<u>Awesome stir-fry</u>

- ½ cup of canola oil
- Low-sodium soy sauce or amino acid
- Baby carrots
- Sugar snap peas
- Water chestnuts
- Red bell peppers, sliced in strips
- Scallions (just the green parts), sliced on a thin bias
- Angel-hair pasta
- Bean sprouts
- Fresh garlic
- Fresh ginger
- Chicken, beef, or any seafood or tofu you like. Make sure you are wearing gloves when touching any raw protein.

It is best to use a wok to cook this dish. But before you get started, you have to set up your *mise en place*. What does this mean? It is fancy chef talk that means to make sure you have everything in place and ready to go. You need to be prepared to work quickly.

- Cut the chicken, or your choice of protein, into bite-size pieces.
- Make sure everything has been washed and dried, especially the bean sprouts.
- Get the oil hot over medium heat, just until it is starting to simmer.

- Add your chicken, let it simmer for a bit, and then add the snow peas.
- You need to do things in the order that it takes to cook each ingredient fully.
- Next, add the carrots and the water chestnuts.
- While that is cooking, boil the pasta until it is al dente, which means "to the tooth."
- Add bean sprouts, and toss.
- Grate the ginger and the garlic into the pan.
- Add the cooked pasta. Toss the whole dish together.
- Add soy or amino acid to the wok; toss it one more time.
- Serve it in warm bowls.
- For a special touch, serve it with sesame seeds and extra soy sauce.
- You will be the best host/hostess ever!

Stuffed potatoes

This serves four people.

- 8 large, raw firm potatoes, all the same size
- 1 medium onion
- A little stale bread, crust removed
- 1 clove fresh garlic
- 1 glass of milk
- 5½ cups minced meat (I use diced ham from the local grocery.)
- A few sprigs of fresh parsley (get flat leaf, not the curly type)
- 8 small slices bacon, smoked or unsmoked, according to your taste

- Butter
- Salt and pepper
- Be sure to wash them off first, and peel them. Cut off one side so it will sit flat in a pan. Cut the top third of the potato; gently scoop the inside out, being careful not to puncture the bottom.
- Break up the bread into small pieces, and soak them in milk. I know it sounds goofy, but now, you need to wring out the moisture.
- Peel and chop the onion and garlic.
- Mix it all together: the meat, onion, garlic, and bread.
- Add the salt, pepper, and parsley.
- Fill the potatoes with the stuffing, and then return the tops.
- Wrap the potatoes with the bacon and put them in a generously buttered baking dish.
- Put the pan in a preheated oven at 400° Fahrenheit (F) for 1 hour and 15 minutes.

Serve while still hot, and offer extra butter, real bacon bits, and real cheddar cheese.

Let's talk pork!

Pork has a love-hate relationship with some people (which I can't understand). I hope that all of you enjoy this recipe.

Roast ham cooked in its own rind

- This recipe serves up to 15 people. You will need a ham that weighs 11.25 pounds in its skin. Ask the butcher to remove the bone.
- Using a very sharp knife, make shallow incisions in the rind, being careful to only cut the rind. Avoid cutting the meat.

- Make a longitudinal cut in the rind.
- Bake in the oven at 350° F for about 4 hours.
- Make sure to baste it with the juice that it is releasing.
- When it is finished, remove the fat cap, and slice the meat into pieces, not too thin and not too thick.
- Serve with the juices drizzled over the meat.

Also serve it with some garlic mashed potatoes or the glazed carrots from the previous recipe.

Now more pork! Woo-hoo!
Loin of pork a la boulangère for six; this means "pork over scalloped potatoes."

- Brush a 3 lb. 5 oz. loin of pork with extra-virgin olive oil and salt, pepper, and some lemon-pepper seasoning.
- Cook in the oven at 450° F. Pull this out right before it is finished, at least five minutes.
- Put in foil to let it finish cooking so it doesn't dry out while the potatoes are cooking.
- Meanwhile, peel 7 oz. of sweet onion, and 1¾ lbs. of potatoes; then, slice them into fairly thick pieces.
- Season the veggies with salt and pepper, and then put them in the oven at 350° F.
- When it is all finished, slice the pork thin, and serve over the potatoes. Spoon the juices from the pork. Finish the dish with salt and pepper and fresh, diced Italian parsley.

Where's the beef?
It is right here…

There are several ways to cook beef:

- Rare only takes about 45 seconds on each side. The meat should be very supple when you press on it with your finger.
- The most common way to cook a steak is medium rare. This means the means that the meat is hot and brown on the outside but barely cooked on the inside. When it is pressed, it is supple but slightly resistant.
- Well-done meat is cooked much longer, up to 7 or 8 minutes on each side. The interior is still fairly red, but the outer edge is dark brown. When pressed, the meat resists noticeably.
- Very well-done meat is totally cooked and strongly resists any pressure. When cut open, the interior is uniformly brown; unfortunately, even the best meat can end up dry when cooked like this.

<u>Roast beef</u>

- Preheat the oven for 20 minutes at 445° F. I think that it is best to truss the roast so it cooks evenly. Put the roast into in a well-oiled (with canola oil) roasting pan. Then, baste it with canola oil, salt, pepper, and a little dried thyme. For more flavor, put some peeled garlic around the roast.
- Cook for 12 to 15 minutes per pound for medium rare. Once you have obtained an internal temperature of 145° F, remove the meat from the roasting pan. Cover the roast in foil so it keeps warm while you deglaze the pan.
- To deglaze the pan, remove it from the heat so you can pour in a bit of red wine. Then, return to heat. Be sure to scrape the goodies from the bottom. That is where all the flavors live.

- Remove the strings from the foil. Cut into thin slices, against the grain.
- Place it on a platter, and then spread the deglazed juices over the roast and vegetables. Serve piping hot. *Enjoy your hard work!*

On to the chicken!
We will start with a simple chicken broth.

- You can start with a whole chicken, but I feel like it turns out better when you start with a boned chicken. It will make a better broth.
- Skim the fat from the carcass, and add 6 cups of water.
- Chop up some vegetables, like ¾ cup of onions, peeled and cut in half. Then, chop 3 carrots, 2 cloves, 2 leeks, coarse salt, 10 peppercorns, some thyme, and some bay leaves.
- All this goes into the pot with the chicken carcass.
- Let this all simmer for 2 hours, skimming off the fat regularly.
- Run the broth through a skimmer to separate the bones and veggies from the broth.
- You can use hot broth to make some chicken-noodle soup or chicken and dumplings. The options are endless.
- If you aren't going to use the broth right away, you can put it a tightly sealed container. It will freeze well in a well-sealed container.

It is handy to make because you can use it in many recipes at any time.

Many people like fish and seafood.
There are many types of fish. Many people don't realize how many types of fish there are. Fish can be divided into a few types:

29

- Round fish swim in vertical positions and have eyes on both sides of their heads.
- Flat fish have asymmetrical, compressed bodies and swim in horizontal positions. Their eyes are on the tops of their heads.
- Flatfish are bottom-feeders and are found in deep ocean waters around the world. The skin on the tops of their bodies is dark, so they can be camouflaged from predators. Their scales and their dorsal fins are small and can change colors according to their surroundings.

Not to forget there are mollusks, such as univalves. Then, there are bivalves, which have two shells, such as clams, oysters, and mussels. Squid and octopus are called cephalopods. They do not have hard outer shells; rather, they have single, thin, internal shells called pens or cuttlebones.

Crustaceans are also shellfish. They have hard outer skeletons, or shells. Crustaceans include lobsters, crabs, and shrimp. The flesh of the fish and shellfish consists primarily of water, protein, fat, and minerals. Fish flesh is composed of short muscle fibers, pleated in shape and separated by delicate connective tissues. Unlike the connective tissue in meat, the connective tissue of fish and shellfish is weak and does not require long cooking times to break it down.

Fish, as well as most shellfish, are naturally tender, so the purpose of cooking is to firm proteins and enhance flavor. The absence of the oxygen-carrying protein myoglobin makes fish very light or white in color. The orange color of fish like salmon and some trout comes from their food.

Compared to meats, fish do not contain large amounts of intermuscular fat. Fish containing a relatively large amount of fat, such as salmon and mackerel, are known as fatty fish. Fish such as cod and haddock, as well as shellfish, are considered lean fish.

Identifying fish and shellfish properly can be difficult because of the vast number of similar-appearing fish and shellfish that separate species within each family. Adding to the confusion are the various colloquial names used or the fact that the same names are given to different fish in different localities. Fish with unappealing names may also be given catchier names for marketing purposes. Moreover, some species are referred to by a foreign name, especially on menus.

The FDA published the *FDA Guide to Acceptable Market Names for Food Fish Sold in Interstate Commerce* in 2009. The list is updated regularly and is available on the FDA's website at the Center for Food. This book attempts to use the most common names for each item, whether they are zoologically accurate or not.

The book discusses round and flat fish and mollusks. Here are a few recipes.

Sautéed halibut with three-color peppers and Spanish olives

- Mise en place: Peel and slice 3 oz. onions, 3 oz. sliced green peppers, 3 oz. sliced red bell peppers, and 3 oz. yellow bell pepper.
- 8 oz. tomato paste
- 2 tsp. of minced garlic
- Spanish olives
- Thyme, fresh if you can find it, otherwise dried
- Lemon juice, 2 fl. Oz.
- Fish stock (If you don't have any, use veggie stock.)
- Season 4 halibut filets with salt and pepper.
- Put the olive oil into a pan large enough to hold 4 full-sized pieces of halibut.
- Sauté the filets until they get a little bit of color; turn once, and then put them in foil so they can stay warm.

- Add the onions and the garlic and sauté for a minute; then add the bell peppers and sauté for 2 minutes.
- Add the tomato, olives, and thyme.
- Add the tomatoes.
- Add the lemon juice and stock to deglaze the pan.
- Return the filets to the pan so the meat can reheat.

Once you have the fish plated, spoon some leftover sauce in the pan over the plated fish. Reseason with salt, pepper, and extra lemon juice. Serve hot.

How about some blue crab cakes?

- As always, you have to do your mise en place.
- 1 lb. crabmeat (Blue is preferred, but if you can't find it, no big deal.)
- 6 fl. Oz. heavy cream
- 2 oz. each red and green bell peppers
- 1 bunch of green onion, finely chopped
- 1 Tbsp. Dijon mustard
- Clarified butter as needed
- Worcestershire sauce to taste
- Tabasco sauce to taste
- 1 egg, slightly beaten
- Carefully pick through the crabmeat, removing any pieces of shell. Keep the lumps of crabmeat as long as possible.
- Place the cream in a saucepan, and bring to a boil. Reduce by about half. Chill the cream well.
- Sauté the bell peppers in a small amount of the clarified butter until tender.

- Combine the crabmeat, reduced cream, bell peppers, green onions, approximately 3 oz. of the bread crumbs, salt and pepper, Dijon mustard, Worcestershire sauce, and tabasco sauce. Mix everything together, keeping the lumps of crab as intact as possible.
- Put the leftover crumbs in a well-greased baking pan (large enough to hold 15 cakes).
- Using a 2-oz. mold, press the patties into even rounds.
- Heat a sauté pan that is large enough to fry a few cakes at a time.
- Use enough clarified butter to cover the bottom of the pan.
- Over moderate heat, brown both sides of each cake; once they are all brown, transfer them to the prepared baking pan.
- Put the cakes on the baking pan.
- Cook in the oven until you are sure they are done.
- Use your meat thermometer to ensure that it reaches over 165° F. Serve hot with tartar sauce or malt vinegar.

Boiled lobster

- 1 lb. 8 oz. lobster
- 4 gallons boiling, salted water
- 4 lemons, cut into wedges
- 2 oz. melted butter
- Drop the lobster into the water. Bring the water back to a boil; reduce to a simmer, and cook the lobster for approximately 12 minutes. Remove the lobster from the pot, strain off the water, and serve immediately with the butter and lemon wedges.

Ceviche

- 1 lb. raw scallops or shrimp and some whitefish, cut coarsely but evenly
- 8 fl. Oz. fresh lime juice
- 2 serrano chilies, minced
- 4 oz. red onions, finely diced
- 6 oz. fresh cilantro, minced
- 8 oz. tomato juice
- 4 Tbsp. olive oil
- 2 tsp. minced garlic
- Salt and pepper to taste
- Chop the scallops, shrimp, and fish evenly and coarsely.
- Place in a nonreactive bowl; add the lime juice.
- Cover and marinate in the refrigerator for 4 hours. The fish should turn opaque and become firm.
- Toss in the remaining ingredients and season with the salt and pepper to taste.

Serve with tortillas or as a salad. If the ceviche is going to be held for more than 2 hours, drain the liquid, and refrigerate separately. The reserved liquid can be tossed in with the other ingredients at service time.

Eggs and breakfast

There are different parts to an egg. There is the albumin, better known as the egg white; and there are the chalazae cords, which are the thick, twisted strings of egg whites that connect the white to the yolk—they are neither imperfections nor embryos. The more prominent the chalazae, the fresher the egg is. Eggs are sold in jumbo, large, medium, small, and peewee sizes.

Grading:
Eggs are graded by the USDA or state according to the same rules. They are graded as follows:

- Grades AA, A, or B means that egg stays fairly compact and spreads slightly.
- Eggs should be a thick, firm white. Storage should be in a cooler that keeps the eggs at a temperature below 45° F. If not, they will go bad quickly.
- Spread should remain compact, but will increase as the quality of the egg goes down.
- The albumin should be clear and thick and should have a prominent chalaza.
- The yolk should be firm and centered. It should stand round and high and be free of damage.
- The shell should be clean, of a normal egg, and unbroken.

Eggs can be cooked in several different ways. They can be poached, fried, and made into omelets. We will start with the easiest ways to cook eggs.

Scrambled eggs (Everyone can do that, right?)

- 12 eggs (more or fewer, depending on how many people are eating)
- 2 fl. Oz. heavy cream
- Salt and pepper to taste

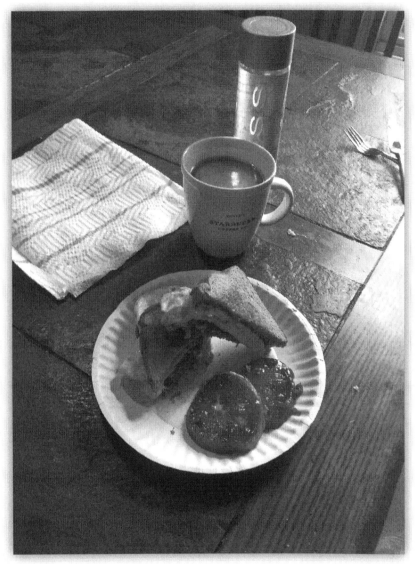

Eggs, bacon, Swiss sandwich with Heirloom tomatoes and a good
cup of coffee

- Clarified butter
- Combine the eggs, cream, salt, and pepper in a mixing bowl. Whisk everything together. Heat the butter in a sauté pan.
- Pour the mixture into the hot pan. Stir frequently. As the eggs begin to set, slowly stir the mixture with a spatula. Lift cooked portions to allow the uncooked eggs to flow underneath. Sprinkle the additional ingredients, such as cheese or herbs. The eggs should be set but still shiny and moist. Remove from the pan, and serve immediately.

Preparing folded omelets

- Fully cook any meats and/or any other vegetables that will be important in your omelet.
- Pour however many eggs you wish into a warm pan with clarified butter. Let them sit, and stir. Add in the ingredients and the cheese.
- Fold one side into the center and the other side over that side to make a perfect pocket.
- Slide onto a prepared plate. Spoon any extra ingredients and cheeses over the omelet. Serve immediately.

Poached eggs

- Water as needed
- 1 tsp. salt
- 1 fl. Oz. vinegar
- 2 eggs
- Bring the water to a simmer; add salt and vinegar.
- Crack one egg into a greased ramekin and drop the eggs in, one by one.

- Cook the eggs to the point at which they are solid, but they're runny on the inside.
- Serve immediately. To make it even more special, serve it with toast.

How about some pancakes?
We will start with buttermilk pancakes.

- 1 lb. flour
- 2 Tbsp. sugar
- 2 oz. buttermilk
- 1 Tbsp. baking powder
- 2 oz. unsalted butter
- 3 eggs, beaten
- Clarified butter, as needed
- Sift the flour, sugar, baking powder, and salt together.
- Combine the buttermilk, melted butter, and eggs.
- Add the wet ingredients to the dry, and mix well.
- Coat the griddle with butter. At 350° F, drop the pancakes in 2 fl. Oz. portions, using a ladle.
- When bubbles start to form on the surface and the crust is starting to brown, flip the cakes over to finish cooking.
- Serve hot with butter and syrup. If you're craving blueberries, you can rinse and dry some; then, add them to the batter, and cook them just like the ones right above this recipe.

How about some crepes?

- 6 whole eggs
- 6 egg yolks
- 12 fl. Oz. water

- 18 fl. Oz. milk
- 6 oz. granulated sugar
- 1 tsp. salt
- 14 oz. flour
- 5 oz. melted butter
- Clarified butter, as needed
- Whisk together the eggs, the egg yolks, water, and milk.
- Stir in the sugar, salt, melted butter, and flour. Whisk everything together. Cover, and set aside to rest for at least an hour.
- Heat a small sauté or crepe pan; brush lightly with the clarified butter. Pour in 1 fl. Oz. batter; swirl to cover the bottom of the pan evenly.
- Cook the crepe until set and light brown, approximately 30 seconds. Flip over, and cook a few seconds longer. Remove from the pan. Repeat this process until the batter is all cooked.
- Cooked crepes may be used immediately or covered and held in a warm oven. Crepes can be wrapped well and refrigerated for 2–3 days or frozen for several weeks.

Staying with breakfast, let's talk about cereals. Oats, rice, and wheat are perhaps the most widely eaten breakfast foods. I personally can't leave out toast! Processed breakfast cereals are cold food made out of these grains. Oatmeal served as "hot porridge" is still popular, especially with toppings such as cream, brown sugar, and fresh or dried fruit. Grits are made from ground corn and are another grain product served hot at breakfast. Grits may be topped with butter and presented as a side dish or served in a bowl like porridge, with cream and brown sugar.

Let's make granola!
You will need the following:

- 8 oz. brown sugar
- 4 fl. Oz. hot water
- 6 fl. Oz. canola oil
- 18 oz. old-fashioned oats
- 2½ oz. coconut, shredded
- 4 oz. wheat germ
- Salt (optional)
- 2 oz. whole wheat flour
- 2 oz. amaranth flour
- 2 oz. unbleached, all-purpose flour
- 2 oz. yellow cornmeal
- 4 oz. chopped pecans
- Dissolve the brown sugar in the hot water. Add the oil.
- Combine all the dry ingredients.
- Add the brown sugar and water to the dry ingredients.
- Spread the granola in a thin layer pan. Bake the granola at 200° F until crisp. Toss lightly with a metal spatula every 30 minutes.
- Cool completely to room temperature, and add some chopped, dried fruit, additional nuts, or fresh fruits when serving. It is also great over yogurt. Take the rest of it, and store it in an airtight container.

Breakfast beverages

If you are anything like me, I can't go through a day without at least four cups of coffee or two espressos. Needless to say, I tend to bounce off the wall.

Coffee begins as the fruit of a small tree grown in tropical and subtropical regions. The fruit, referred to as the cherry, is bright red. The cherries are harvested by hand and then cleaned, fermented, and hulled, leaving the green coffee beans. The beans are then roasted to any degree of darkness, ground to any degree of fineness, and brewed in any number of ways.

Only two species of coffee are routinely used: arabica and robusta. Arabica beans are the most important commercially and the ones from which the finest coffees are produced. Robusta beans do not produce as flavorful a drink as arabica. Nevertheless, robusta beans are becoming increasingly significant commercially, in part because they are healthier and more fertile than arabica. The conditions in which the beans are grown have almost as much effect on the final product as subsequent roasting, grinding, and the air; the beans' origin is critical to the product's final quality. Roasting releases and enhances the flavors of the coffee.

There are several ways to roast coffee:

- City roast, also called American or brown roast. City roast is the most widely used in most American cafés.
- Brazilian is somewhat darker than city roast. This roast should present a dark-roast flavor. The flavor should present a slight taste of oil.
- Viennese is also known as medium-dark roast. Viennese roast is generally between a city roast and a French roast.
- French roast, also called a New Orleans or dark roast, approaches an espresso without sacrificing smoothness. The beans should be the color of semisweet chocolate, with apparent oiliness on the surface.
- Espresso roast, also known as Italian, is the darkest of all. The beans are roasted until they are virtually burnt. The beans should be black and oily.

Now onto my favorites: making bread and cheese! Yes, from scratch!

Owning an Italian restaurant, I prepared focaccia every morning. It has to proof several times a day. Bear with me; everything I say may sound convoluted. This will fill a sheet pan measuring 18 by 13 inches by 1 inch thick.

- 2 cups plus 2 oz. water
- 1 tsp. yeast
- 1 tsp. sugar
- 2 oz. olive oil
- 5½ cups of flour
- 1 tsp. salt
- Mix the water, sugar, olive oil, flour, and (always last) the salt. If the salt goes in earlier, it will kill the yeast. Mix it all together by hand. Make sure your hands are well oiled. Knead the dough in a well-oiled mixing bowl fixed with a hook. Put in a well-oiled bowl. Cover the dough with a well-oiled film. Let it sit undisturbed for at least 75 minutes.
- Once it has doubled in size, take it out, and press it onto a well-greased pan, preferably a pan covered with parchment paper. Punch down with your fingers to make dimples. Proof for 1 hour. Stretch to the corners. Proof for 30 minutes. Bake at 450° F for 30 minutes.
- Check in on it every 15 minutes.
- 15 minutes before it is done baking, baste with garlic butter, and add the herbs of your choice. I would recommend dried parsley, dried oregano, and even sunflower seeds. And in the last few minutes, add some mozzarella cheese. Cut into 4 × 4-inch squares. Either serve it as bread for a sandwich, or cut it into small strips, and serve them with marinara sauce, olive oil, or some homemade garlic oil.

How about fresh pizza dough?

Good news: No metric measures! This recipe will make 2 or 3 medium pizzas.

- 3 cups cool water
- 1 Tbsp. yeast
- 3 Tbsp. sugar
- 3 Tbsp. olive oil
- 6–7 cups bread flour
- 1 Tbsp. salt
- Let the dough rest for 15–20 minutes in a well-oiled bowl; separate the dough into 2–3 even balls; let it rest for 15–20 minutes.
- Once they have doubled in size, take the balls of dough out, and put them on an oiled sheet pan.
- Pat the dough into even circles, and let them rest on well-oiled sheet pans.
- Add the basic ingredients: tomato sauce, green peppers, meat if you please, mushrooms, and cheese.
- Bake in the oven on a pizza stone at 400° F for 20 minutes. Check on them to make sure the cheese is melted and the crust isn't burning.
- When it is ready to come out, let it rest after it comes out. If you try to cut it right out of the oven, the cheese will ooze out too early. Cut it, serve it hot, and serve it with some condiments, such as crushed red peppers, garlic powder, pepperoncini, artichoke, parmesan cheese, and extra tomatoes—maybe some salt and pepper to taste.

How about some homemade bagels?

We at Vecchio's made "bagel bombs." What's that? It is a round bagel stuffed with cream cheese and some smoked salmon (if you like).

You will need…

- 1100 grams bread flour
- 2¼ tsp. yeast
- 3½ cups water
- 2 Tbsp. salt
- Throw everything in a mixing bowl.
- Mix until well combined (3–5 minutes).
- Put into a well-oiled bowl, and let it rest in the fridge for at least an hour.
- Take this time to make your mix: a filling of cream cheese, bacon, chives, or any kind of fillings you might like on your bagel.
- Make sure your cream cheese is soft enough to spread.
- Take the "bomb" dough out, and spread it into 8 even rounds.
- Spoon the rounds with the filling, and wrap them back into a ball. Put on an egg wash and then add some extra seasonings, such as dried parsley, dried oregano, or poppy seeds. If you really like cheese, add some mozzarella cheese to the top as well. Bake in a 400° F oven for 8–10 minutes. Don't be alarmed. They may bust—hence the name "bagel bombs."
- Serve hot; just be careful, as they will be very hot, especially the center. I would suggest a nice cup of coffee, tea, or even some orange juice. Also have a fruit salad. That will make it "healthy," right?

More bread if you like?

Let's make some bread bowls! This will make 8 bowls. It's better if you make the soup yourself.

You need the following:

- ¼ tsp. yeast
- 1¼ cup warm water
- 1 Tbsp. olive oil
- 3½ cups bread flour
- In a big bowl, mix the warm water with the yeast and sugar in the bowl. Whisk the combination until it is fully mixed. Let it stand until it becomes frothy and looks creamy.
- Add the flour, 1 cup at a time. Add the salt. Continue to mix by hand once the dough has come together.
- Pour out the dough onto a well-floured sheet.
- Knead the dough until it is smooth, about 6 or 7 minutes. Put the dough in a well-oiled bowl, turn it over, and add more oil to it. Then, cover it with a clean, damp cloth, and let it sit in a warm place in your house for about 40 minutes.
- Preheat the oven to 400° F. Once the loaf has proofed, divide it into 4 large loaves. In a small bowl, beat together an egg white and 1 Tbsp. of water, and brush the loaves. Put them in the oven. Bake for 10–15 minutes; baste again with the remaining egg yolks and water. Bake them again for another 10–15 minutes. Let them cool on a cooling rack. Once they are cool, cut a piece of the top off to make a lid.
- Scoop out the center, leaving a ¾-inch shell around the bowls. Fill the bowl with hot soup, replace the lid, and serve hot.

<u>As much as I love making bread…</u>
I love making homemade pasta and cheese. But I found a recipe by Frank's mom from 1950. It is Mom's famous manicotti that you can make at home.

Here is what you need:

- 1 pint part-skim ricotta cheese
- 8 oz. shredded mozzarella cheese
- ¾ cup Parmesan cheese
- 2 eggs
- 1 tsp. dried parsley
- Salt to taste
- Ground black pepper
- 1 jar spaghetti sauce
- 5½ oz. manicotti noodles
- Cook manicotti in boiling water until it's done. Drain and rinse in *cold* water.
- Preheat the oven to 350° F.
- In a large bowl, combine the ricotta, mozzarella, and ½ cup of the Parmesan, dried parsley, eggs, and salt and pepper.
- Pour half of the sauce into a 12 × 17–inch baking dish.
- Fill the manicotti with 3 Tbsp. of the cheese mixture, and arrange over the sauce. Pour the rest of the sauce and Parmesan over the top.
- Bake 45 minutes, or until bubbly.
- Serve hot, and *always* put extra seasonings, such as Parmesan cheese, fresh oregano, parsley, or basil on the table.

Here are the food safety rules, according to the Food Safety government website:

- Ground meat, beef, pork, veal, lamb, steaks, roasts, and pork chops: Between the temperatures of 160–165° F.
- Poultry, such as chicken, turkey, duck, and goose; stuffing; leftovers; and casseroles: Internal temperature 165° F for everything.

- Eggs: Cook until the eggs and yolk are firm. Egg products, cook to 160° F.
- Fish is a little more confusing.
- Fin fish: Cook to 140° F or until flesh is opaque and separates easily with a fork.
- Shrimp, lobster, and crabs: Cook until flesh is pearly and opaque.
- Clams, oysters, mussels: Cook until the shells open on their own.
- Scallops: Cook until flesh is milky white or opaque and firm.

Now, some recipes for my vegetarian friends!

We will start with dauphine potatoes, which are prepared by mixing mashed potatoes with a choux pastry mix. Choose firm, white, smooth-skinned potatoes.

Peel and wash 1¾ pounds of potatoes, and cook in salted and lightly oiled water. Once they are cooked, drain the water. Make sure that they are totally dry. Press them through a potato press to make sure they are completely smooth.

Time to prepare your choux.

- 1 generous cup milk, 2 oz. butter, and 1 tsp. salt
- Heat the mixture, being sure not to burn it or allow it to scorch.
- Add 2 beaten eggs.
- Gradually let the mixture cool.
- Form the potatoes into bite-size pieces.
- Return the potatoes to the choux in the pan, and toss the potatoes together.
- Put the mixture in a greased pan. Mix the whole dish evenly.

- Add the mixed potatoes to the dish, and add any types of cheese and herbs of your liking to the dish.
- Bake the mix in the oven at 350° F for at least 45 minutes.
- Serve hot, and provide extra salt, pepper, cheese, and dried parsley. Serve with juice or even mimosas. You will be the best host/hostess *ever*!

I said that I loved making bread…but I really love making cheese and pasta!

I used to teach pasta and cheese classes around the local round here in southern Indiana. I'll begin with pasta. The reason that I started with pasta is that it is easier to explain and easier to do at home. The ingredients are easy to find.

I will start with the different types of pasta.

<u>Long strands:</u>

- Spaghetti: Match with meaty tomato, creamy seafood, broth, or olive oil–based sauces. The earthy flavor and rough texture of whole wheat or spelt spaghetti pair well with chunky, country-style sauces, especially ones containing mushrooms or green bell peppers. A spaghetti made of rice flour is more delicate and will fall apart easily if overcooked. Toss with olive oil or broth-based sauce, herbs, or spring vegetables.
- Spaghettini: This is slightly thinner and more delicate than spaghetti. Pair with broth, olive oil, or light tomato sauces.
- Vermicelli: Thinner than spaghettini, this will be overwhelmed by thick, heavy sauces. Use lighter tomato, olive oil, or light broth-based sauces.

- Angel hair: It cooks quickly, often in just two minutes. It's great in lighter entrées or side dishes, or when broken up for soups. Use with thin tomato or broth-based sauces, or toss with olive oil, finally chopped cooked vegetables, and shrimp.
- Bucatini: A hollow strand that pairs well with thicker sauces.

Ribbon Strips:
The following types can measure up to several inches wide.

- Linguini: Both white or clam sauces are traditional with this $1/16$-inch-wide pasta. But linguini marries with almost any sauce.
- Fettuccine: This ⅛-inch-wide noodle is classically paired with a creamy Alfredo sauce, but any sauce with a medium-to-thick consistency is good.
- Tagliatelle: These are wider than fettuccine and are traditionally paired with meat or light fish sauces or pesto.
- Pappardelle: These one-inch-wide noodles match with hearty meat, cream, and vegetable sauces. In Tuscany, they're served with wine-and-tomato duck or rabbit sauces.
- Lasagna: This is a familiar noodle about 2 inches wide with curly edges. The no-boil variety has straight edges. If using this, don't be tempted to cook evenly briefly. Noodles will stick together and become almost impossible to separate. Have a little sauce or broth on hand, or even a bit of water to drizzle around the edges, which may become dry.

Tubular Pastas:
These are usually 2–3 inches long, with a center hole ranging from a half inch to 1 inch wide. All of these are perfect for baked dishes.

- Rigatoni: Short, fat tubes with ridges on the edges on the exterior can be paired with hearty meat sauces or chunky vegetable sauces of eggplant, tomatoes, and bell peppers. Thick tomato or cream-based sauces work well.
- Penne: These are short, hollow tubes that are cut diagonally. Penne rigate have ribbed surfaces, whereas penne lisce are smooth. These can go with a wide range of sauces, from meat to cheese to those with vinaigrette sauces.
- Ziti: This medium-sized tube is slightly curved and pairs well with any hearty tomato, cheese, or roasted-vegetable-based sauce.
- Manicotti: These large tubes can be filled with meat, cheese, seafood, or vegetable filling. Cannelloni filling can also be used in manicotti.

Molded Shapes:

These shapes capture sauce in their grooves and can be paired with the same kinds of sauces as tube-shaped pastas.

- *Conchiglie* or shells: Choose any tiny shape for soups or medium-size shape for baked dishes or other entrées, salads, and side dishes. Large shells can be stuffed with meat, cheese, or vegetable filling and baked.
- Cavatappi: This pasta is formed in a spiral-tube shape. It is known by other names, usually rigati (lines or grooves on the outside surface of the pasta).
- Farfalle (bowties or butterflies): The pasta is cut into squares and then pinched in the center to make the distinctive shape. It can be difficult to get the center to cook, so it should be tested repeatedly for tenderness. Even so, the center will probably be a little chewy. Pair with creamy béchamel-based sauces, or toss in olive oil, herbs, and finely diced vegetables.

- Orecchiette: This round, thumbprint-shaped pasta is often paired with vegetable- or broth-based sauces or with vegetables, such as broccoli rabe, that have been lightly cooked in olive oil.
- Fusilli: The twisted shape is great for salads, side dishes, and entrées because it pairs very well with any sauce. A flavorful pesto is a wonderful choice.
- *Radiatore*: This is a fun shape with ruffled edges that marries well with most sauces and zesty vinaigrettes.

<u>Soups and side dishes</u>
Tiny pastas that kids love, including the alphabet, stars, and tiny butterflies, are great for kids.

- Orzo: A small, rice-shaped pasta for soups, salads, or quick side dishes. Use with lighter sauces.
- *Acini pepe*: If you were to cut a dry piece of spaghetti into 1/16-inch pieces, you'd have the approximate size of this pasta. Toss it into soups, or serve as a side dish instead of rice.
- *Fregola sarda*: These tiny, rough-textured balls have been toasted and are wonderful cooked in broth and tossed with chopped herbs and fine shreds of cheese.
- Ditalini: This means "little thimbles" in Italian, and the pasta is most typically used in the Campania region of Italy, where it is found in *pasta e fagioli*, minestrone, and other classic soups—even a simple bowl of plain broth.

Sources: *Cook's Illustrated Italian Classics*; *Bugialli on Pasta*, by Giuliano Bugialli

Now, let's talk about rice!

Rice is a wonderful ingredient. It can be used in many ways: rice for breakfast, pilaf, risotto, sushi, and so many things.

I will start with some of my favorites to make. It is important to know what type of dish you would like to prepare. I know it sounds picky, but this affects how much water you need to make your dish. The more water you use, the looser the dish is. The less you use, the stickier the rice will be.

For the perfect breakfast or soup dish, you need plenty of salted and buttered water. Cook plenty of the rice for 10–15 minutes or until it is chewy, but not falling apart. Drain, but hang onto the water. (It is great if you have an upset stomach, as I did while I was recovering from my liver transplant.) Anyhow, take the warm rice, add some butter and sugar, and serve in a bowl. If you are making soup, sauté some carrots, onions, and green peppers. Then, place the drained rice in a pot of warm broth with the carrots, peppers, and celery, and warm through. Serve with warm bread and a nice sparkly beverage.

If you are craving pilaf, I have a great recipe to share.

<u>Pilaf with clams</u>

- Use long-grain rice.
- Sauté some whole, peeled garlic and some onions in olive oil and a pat of butter; if you like it spicy, add some crushed red pepper.
- Scrub the clams thoroughly to ensure they don't have any sand in them. Make sure that you are using a large pot.
- Add 2 cups of chicken broth and 2 cups of rice. Bring to a boil; add in the veggies; add the clams, and cook until they open.
- Plate in warm bowls, and make sure you have a ton of napkins.

Italian risotto

To make an authentic Italian risotto, you need a special type of rice. You can use one of the following: Arborio, Carnaroli, Vialone Nano. They are short, thick grains that have a high level of starch, and if they are prepared without overboiling the rice, its distinctive character is assured. Risotto should be creamy but not sticky, with every grain tender.

- Over low heat, brown 1 sliced onion, 2 cloves chopped garlic, and 1 Tbsp. tomato sauce with virgin olive oil in a fairly large, flat-bottomed skillet.
- Add 1¼ cups rice, and sauté it for 5 minutes, stirring with a wooden spoon until the grains are entirely coated and turn opaque. Meanwhile, heat 3 cups of homemade chicken broth in another pan.
- Then, add ⅓ cup plus 1½ Tbsp. dry white wine. Then, add half of the chicken broth, followed by salt, pepper, and dried oregano, all in the same pan.
- Cook the rice over low heat until the liquid is absorbed; then, add the rest of the broth. Make sure that the texture is correct: not too runny and not too stiff. When you are happy, serve it in a warm bowl with a dash of fresh, grated Parmesan cheese and a chiffonade of basil.

Lasagna

When you make lasagna, buy fresh noodles if you can. Well, if you are brave enough, make them yourself.

- Check your fresh lasagna to make sure it is uniform in color, with no pale patches. If you find some, discard them.

- Boil plenty of salted water over high heat, and add some olive oil.
- Make sure that you shake the flour off the noodles so it doesn't make the final product a big ball of dough.
- When the water is at a hard boil, plunge the pieces of pasta in 2 by 2 so they don't stick to each other.
- Monitor the cooking process carefully, as its time will vary according to the volume of water.
- Take a piece out of the pasta, and taste it.

You can use it in several different ways, including the way we are used to—stacked with cheese, meat, and sauce. I would suggest you would use dried pasta for this preparation, because it is much stronger. For this particular recipe, I would use a light sauce, such as a light lemon, chive, or olive oil sauce. You can also cut it up in triangles and spread it with some strawberry jelly, some fresh-cut strawberries, and lemon slices.

I love fresh ravioli!

Go buy some fresh lasagna, cut it into ravioli squares, and put a damp cloth over them, because you are about to make your own cheese—*yes*, you are going to make your cheese.

Ricotta is originally made from the whey from leftover mozzarella. I make it the easy way. You will need:

- 1 gallon pasteurized whole milk
- 1 tsp. Epsom salt
- A sieve prepared with cheesecloth that has been folded numerous times, until you have 5–6 layers. Place the lined colander over a large bowl.
- Pour the milk into a nonreactive pot (stainless steel works best). Add the Epsom salt. Gradually heat the milk over medium heat.

- Stir frequently, scraping the bottom to ensure that it doesn't scorch.
- As the milk comes to temperature, the curds will begin to form on the surface. Skim as the curds come to the surface. For more wet curds, put them directly into the bowl; for more dry curds, strain them through the colander, which I recommend for this recipe. But don't get rid of the whey.
- Spoon the dry ricotta into the cut ravioli. Use an egg wash to seal the top sheet of the pasta. It helps to use a fork to help seal the pasta. Be careful not to poke the ravioli with the fork, or you will have a mess.
- Bring your salted, oiled water to a rapid boil water over medium heat. Drop the ravioli in very carefully so they don't stick. When they are close to being done, pull them out, and layer them into a well-oiled baking pan. Layer with a light, prewarmed tomato sauce. Bake only until the dish is warmed throughout. Top with Parmesan cheese and some fresh parsley, oregano, or basil.

Saving your ricotta

- Your ricotta will dry out in the refrigerator. If you need it to be more wet, just add a little sour cream or heavy cream, and it will come right back!

Whey-t a minute!!

- Use your whey. Replace the water in pizza dough for a richer pastry. Give to your four-legged friends and family. Many farmers like to use whey to give extra nutrients to their livestock.

Pizza dough made with whey

Prep time: 20 minutes
Cook time: 30 minutes
Total time: 30 minutes
Total time: 50 minutes
Yield: 2 (12 inches) or 1 (14 inch) deep

Ingredients:

- 3 to 3½ cups all-purpose flour
- 1 Tbsp. instant or rapid-rise yeast
- 1 cup warm whey (105–110° F)
- 2 Tbsp. olive oil
- Cornmeal

Preparation:

- In a large bowl, mix the warm whey, yeast, and oil. Let set for 5 minutes so the yeast can "bloom." Gradually mix in flour and salt. Once incorporated, knead for 4–6 minutes. (This process can easily be done in a stand mixer with a dough hook.)
- Let rest on a floured surface for 10 minutes.
- Roll to fit your favorite pan or stone. Sprinkle the pan with cornmeal before placing the dough on it.
- Top the pizza as desired, and bake at 400° F for 20–30 minutes or until done.

Let's make some fresh mozzarella!
Make sure the milk for this cheese is *not ultrapasteurized*!

- Homogenized milk will work fine.
- Fresh-farmed milk will work, but I would encourage you try 1 gallon of store-bought whole milk.
- You can use low-fat milk, but the cheese will be less flavorful and much drier.

You will need:

- A 6–8-quart stainless-steel pot.
- A stainless steel slotted spoon or strong plastic spoon
- A 2-quart microwave safe mixing bowl
- Measuring spoons
- A thermometer that will clearly read 80–120° F

Prepare your work area:

- Do not prepare any other food while you are making cheese.
- Put all food products away.
- Move all food products away.
- Move all sponges, cloths, and dirty towels away from your work surface; wipe your sink and stove with soap and water.
- Finally, use your antibacterial cleaner to wipe down all your surfaces.

Process:

- Crush 1 whole tablet of rennet, and dissolve in ¼ cup of cool, unchlorinated water. Set aside for later.
- Add 1½ tsp. citric acid, diluted in 1 cup of cool water, to 1 gallon of cold milk; stir well. I would put the solution in your

cold pot, and then pour cold milk into your pot quite quickly to mix well with the citric acid. This will bring the milk to the proper acidity to stretch well later.

- Next, heat this milk to 90° F. As you approach 90° F, you may notice your milk starting the curds to separate due to the acidity and temp.
- At 90° F, remove the pot from the burner, and slowly add your rennet (which you prepared in the previous step) to the milk. Stir in a loop in a top-to-bottom motion for approximately 30 seconds; then, stop. Cover the pot, and leave it undisturbed for 5 minutes. I've had it take anywhere from 15 minutes to 2 hours. *Be patient!* Check the curd. If it is too soft, or the whey is milky, let it sit for a few more minutes. It is ready when it cools. Form it into a ball, and drop it into ice water to cool; then, refrigerate.

The water-bath method (my preferred)

Heat a pot to 185° F. Ladle the curds of your mozzarella that are coming to the surface into a cheesecloth-covered colander, folding the curds gently as you drain the whey.

- Dip the curds in the colander into the hot water. After several times, take a spoon, and fold the curds until they start to become elastic and stretchable. This happens when the curd temperature reaches 135° F. It's easier to do in 2 batches.
- When it is stretchable, remove the curd from the liquid, and pull like taffy. This stretching elongates the proteins. If it does not stretch easily, return it to the hot water for more heat.
- At this point add 1 tsp., more or less, of salt and/or fresh herbs and work into the cheese. Stretch the cheese until it is smooth and shiny.

- This is when you shape your cheese. You can make a ball, long balls, bite-size morsels, string cheese, or you can wrap it with prosciutto or roll it with basil.
- When you're finished, submerge it in ice water. This keeps the cheese from getting grainy. Then, you can wrap it in plastic wrap.

Options

- You can make your curds and stretch them later, which I have found to be easier. Just put them in a plastic bag, and then work them in a few days.
- A substitution of reconstituted dry-milk powder and cream is a great option.
- Lipase can be added to your milk to create a more Italian cheese flavor.
- If you want a softer texture, do not let the curds set as firm, and work them less when draining and kneading. This will make a moister cheese.

What happened?

- If your curd looks like ricotta after you've added your rennet and let it set, there could be 1 of 3 problems.
  1. You may be stirring too long after adding the rennet. The milk needs to be *very still* for at least 30–60 seconds.
  2. The label on the on the milk didn't reveal that it was ultrapasteurized.
  3. If your curds won't stretch, put them back in the microwave or water bath. It may just not be hot enough.

- If you find that your cheese is too dry, next time, try the following:
  1. Omit the step after cutting the curd where you heat it to 105–110° F.
  2. Add ¼ tsp. less citric acid to your milk at the beginning of the process.
  3. Stretch it less at the end, and cover it with cold water.

Here is a lesson on some of the terms that you may have never heard:

- Citric acid is naturally found in citrus fruit and is what gives the "sour" flavor. It's also used as a dietary supplement. Locally it can be found at Elbert's Natural Food Market in the "Raw" section. You can find in regular grocery stores. You can find it in the canning section. Look for the Ball company. You can always go online and order it.
- Rennet is an enzyme that is naturally found in a calf's stomach. It was accidentally discovered when people tried to store milk in the stomachs of sheep. It comes both in a liquid or a tablet (which I prefer). You can find it at Whole Foods, but I usually like to order it online. I didn't go over the microwave method, but a lot of people like to do it that way.

OK, OK…enough endless information already!

I have used my mozz for many things. I like to "show off." Don't judge me; you will do the same thing when you start getting credit. Use it in a salad—make a fresh caprese (tomato, fresh mozz, and fresh basil); just drizzle it with some high-quality olive oil or a twenty-five-year-old balsamic vinegar.

The *best* way to showcase your new skills with fresh mozzarella

60

You need:

- Thinly sliced *prosciutto di Parma*
- Fresh mozzarella
- Basil
- Himalayan sea salt
- A good extra-virgin olive oil and 25-year-old balsamic vinegar
- Working quickly, lay a sheet of plastic wrap on the counter to use as a work surface. Lay the warm cheese in a rectangle.
- Working quickly again, layer the prosciutto in a single layer.
- Roll the log, prosciutto on the outside, and put the basil on top; roll tightly, and chill immediately.
- When it is time to serve, cut the roll in ½-inch slices, and serve on crostini. Drizzle with olive oil or vinegar if desired; sprinkle with salt.

Let's change topics altogether…

As I have said in the past, my husband, Dan, is a criminal attorney, and he likes to take me to court. Of course, you should know me well enough by now to know that I sincerely "love" going with him. So I am going to tell you about my day yesterday.

April 26, 2016

Picture this: I am sitting in the law library, stuck in the same seat because he is afraid that I will wander somewhere I shouldn't be. What kind of shit is that? So I am writing this for your entertainment. I should probably shred this before it gets into your hands. No luck. You're welcome!

I am sitting here, looking around, and I see a whole bookshelf of Supreme Court reports. I couldn't help but wonder what they were ruling on. What could I find in these books? And then next to me were rows and rows of treaties. What are treaties for? I didn't get an answer, because it was time to go to court. Yay!

Sometimes I think that I would be a good lawyer. But Big D (my name for my husband) has assured me that is a terrible idea. He says you have to be smart and methodical. OK, that's not me at all. I consider myself very smart, but I'm not methodical at all. If you know me, I am a hothead. You cross me, bend over and kiss my…I tend to fly off the handle.

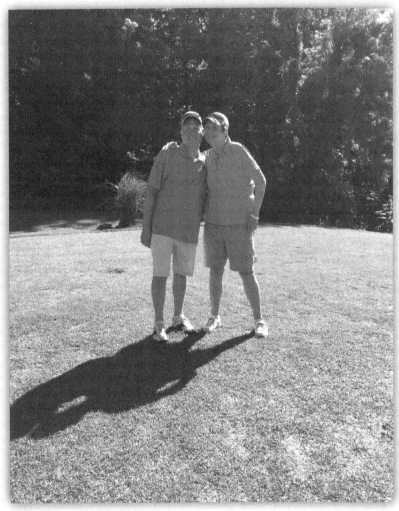

Now I've been moved into the first of three courtrooms. It is the coldest courtroom I've ever been dragged into. It is fucking cold in here. I *love* my husband, but he is sitting in front of me, and I can't help to wonder if he can feel that, at this *very* moment, I am trying to stare a hole through his head. I can't wait to ask him when I can get out of this frozen hell.

This alleged criminal keeps walking by, and he smells exactly like what I expect an alleged criminal would smell like. Thankfully, a very dapper African-American gentleman just walked by. He was a sharp-dressed man, and he smelled like heaven. He kind of reminded me of the guy who played Johnnie Cochran in the O. J. Simpson movie. Then the douchemaster just walked in and went straight up to the judge, passing up everyone in line. Grr. That is another reason that I can't be a lawyer. You can't be the lawyer and the judge. I feel like that is a stupid rule, but I can see that. That is why Dan says there is no place in the courtroom for me. So why does he keep dragging me to these things? It is because I sit in the room and shake my head. And according to Big D, that, too, is unacceptable.

Onto courtroom number two. At least it is warmer—new lawyers, new people. Same alleged criminal smell, and now I smell like smoke. Great.

April 29, 2016

Yeah I know that I skipped a few days, but the next few days were fun days. Well, let me rephrase: the first day was superfun! We decided to go play golf at our favorite course, Cambridge Golf Course, near Evansville, Indiana.

We decided to play twelve holes. No big deal for young folks like us, right? We'll just say that it didn't go like I saw it in our heads. We stopped taking score at hole number five. Who needs to take score if it is just the two of us?

So obviously, we both swung our hearts and butts off. Dan swung more than me, but when I swung, I put my whole body into it. Big D did the same thing. We went to the nineteenth hole (which means the clubhouse restaurant). We splurged on Mountain Dew, loaded buffalo chips, and a twelve-inch pizza. Yum!

About halfway home I started getting a terrible headache, and my face was on fire. Big D had a terrible stomachache, so it was imperative that we got home very quickly. By the time we got home, we both needed to take a shower. I hate smelling like the great outdoors.

For three days after that, we sat on the couch and did nothing but sit on the couch, drink Gatorade, and try not to move. We kept arguing about which of us got to let out our dog, Booker, who wanted to play for fifteen minutes and then take naps for the rest of the day. That was OK with us, because that's all we wanted to do. We went into the bedroom and got on our jammies and then came back to the couch. I spent the rest of the night sitting on the couch. Me typing, Dan playing his computer games. We obviously fell asleep cuddled up on the couch—Dan, Amanda, and Booker all in a small pile. We finally woke up and went to the bedroom, where we all continued to cuddle.

Now let's talk about the following days. The Bookster was all up and running around. We were lying there, wondering who was going to let our playful little dog out. I tried my "I'll give you a dollar if you do it" line. As usual, that didn't work. So I got up and was as sore as I have ever been. And trust me, I've been sore in my days. So by day number three, we were both up and walking with support. My "Boss" should be proud. It turned out to be a great day. Our best friends were closing their winery, so we went down to congratulate them and feast on the cheese, cake, and cupcakes. What a great day! Then we went to Schnuck's and got some salads and some things we needed. Then back to the couch to rest again, ahh…

Three

THREE DAYS IN ARKANSAS WITH THREE (SWEET) OLD LADIES

I had to put the sweet in parentheses because Momma J (Dan's mom, Janice) said I had to put that in so they don't look so bad. She and her sisters invited me to go with them to Arkansas to shop for fabric. Yes, I said fabric. Momma B (Brenda) was pretty calm until we all got to our destination. Prior to meeting up with the sisters, Janice and I went to Burger King to use the restroom and grab a snack, and I saw that they had crowns, so I picked one up to suck up to the sisters. I hadn't met all of them, except during a funeral, so I needed to impress them. So Janice and I went to Debbie's (Momma DJ's) house because she was driving; she had the biggest truck. I later found out that she was the one who was truly crazy.

We went to Batesville, Arkansas. Where is that, you ask? I have no earthly idea. We were in Podunk, Arkansas. No, it doesn't have the scary hotel like in the movies; however, it was a very cool place. I was a little disappointed that I couldn't stay in a haunted hotel. I did, however, die twice, both by vehicle accidents, by two different sisters. Momma DJ "ran out of road." We were tooling along, and she saw the "road closed" sign, and instead of following the traffic, she slammed on the brakes. I screamed, which made everyone else scream. We finally calmed down and went on our way. The second time was when Momma B decided to drive down a one-way street the *wrong* way. I kept telling her that it was wrong, but she just kept saying, "No, Amanda, this is the way to go." Needless to say, I was right. She realized that when a car came barreling down toward us. That is when I got my own "I told you so" moment.

We finally made it! We found a great restaurant called Big. They had the best fresh-cut French fries. The guy was literally cutting them by hand. Delicious. We also had a couple of different types of sandwiches. And of course, all Southern ladies, me included, *need* fried pickles. I put myself in the "Southern ladies club" because I was born in Southern Illinois. I got really pissed because one of the workers at the fabric factory kept calling it "IllINOISE." Then she said, "I thought you were saying, 'I'm annoyed.'"

To this I replied, "Yes, I am annoyed, because I really need to pee."

Then she said, "Just go younder." What the hell is younder? Lucky for her, I made it.

Finally the shopping could begin. Janice and I went one direction, and Momma B and Momma DJ went a different way. We went and found a lot of fun patterns, like rubber duckies and the one where the monkey sees nothing, says nothing, and hears nothing. We bought them for her sisters. Their motto was, "What happens in Arkansas stays in Arkansas." So I'm guessing that they will not want to read this book…heh heh.

So the sisters spent $2,900 on fabric. Yeah, on fabric. They will make more than double on that amount of fabric. They are very talented quilters, and they make things like purses, billfolds, and hats. Momma J makes supercute headbands and flags and embroiders inspirational sayings. She also helps her husband, Frank (my second dad), paint the woodworks that he makes. These include bird and squirrel feeders, bread boxes, shelving, card holders, and soap holders. He also can engrave things in the wood and even on glass. They all sell their items at craft fairs and online.

We ended up having a really good time. Brenda taught me a new saying while trying to fix my hair. Mind you, I am six feet tall, and she…we'll say that she's not. So when she needed me to sit down so she could reach my head, she would look at me and say, "Sit-ye-ass-down."

Janice and I picked out a few fun prints. One was a pattern with rubber duckies. Another had three monkeys. We decided she was going to embroider, "See no evil, say no evil, hear no evil." Pretty catchy, huh? With the duckies, she was going to cut out duck patterns and then sew them onto hand towels. I found a pattern that I'm having made into a purse by Momma B. Now that I reread this, I'm starting to see that I must have had some fun. Shh…

Four

I Won an Award

Yesterday, May 11, 2016, I was invited to my physical therapy alma mater. This facility is named RHI, which is the Rehabilitation Hospital of Indiana. I, along with thirty-one other people, was awarded patient of the year. I didn't realize that they have been doing this since 2013. They have had two to three thousand patients each year. Every year they honor several people who have accomplished their goals for the year to the best of their abilities. I was amazed with the people who were honored. I don't feel like I can even describe the individuals I met.

There were several individuals who had experienced strokes that left them completely paralyzed. Some had TBIs (traumatic brain injuries), which are caused by multiple causes. One gentleman even had a scar on his head from jumping in front of a car to save a lady he had never met. It left him with a scar on his head and in his heart. It was a touching story, which left me speechless. There was another man who was six feet seven and was a well-known basketball star. I was proud to see him standing tall to accept his reward. But at the same time, it broke my heart to hear his story. He got into a car accident that left him unable to walk, talk, or play the game that had made him famous in Indiana.

They finally got to me and began telling the story of my recovery. The gentleman started telling about when I was admitted; I couldn't walk, talk, eat, or speak. It took many weeks of learning to walk with my physical therapist, Bill (my short, sweet physical therapist). He is secretly my hero. The other man in my life who "made sure" that I could walk again is my good buddy, Joe. Joe is six feet three with an infectious personality. In fact, we still work together every week. I am in a program that allows me to work out with peers who have similar abilities. It is a great free program sponsored by one of our local universities. The facility in Indy also started me working with a speech therapist to help me relearn how to speak.

I had lost that ability after my trach. After many weeks I finally started forming words; then came phrases. I got "I love you" for Dan. Then everyone else got, "Shut up and *get out*!" Next, I said, "Oops" on camera, followed by "I'm sorry." At least I got a good laugh. That's OK, right? I got an award and a brick that will be put in the "Pathway to Independence." I was very proud and was tooting my own horn. I honestly know—and knew then—that I was being stupid and selfish. It was just too easy to get caught up in it. I'm truly embarrassed that I would think that I had it any worse than I did.

And then *just* this afternoon, May 16, the Boss put me in my place; she said, "We are going to have fun today. I got new toys this weekend." Yeah, it was a ladder that you put on the floor. Better than having to climb it, right? Nooo way! I had to move from rung to rung, staggering my feet. Then I had to do it backward. Two feet in and then two feet out. And then forward and then all the way back. Greeeaat!

And I got my biggest laugh in a long time. Not me—the people who were watching me trying to jump. She put me on the trampoline and told me not to hold on. The Boss made me hold onto the handles and squat and then jump as high as I could. Needless to say this six-foot-tall body does not like to jump. I got tired of hearing, "Come on, you used to be a volleyball player." Yes, I was, and I was damn good at it. Since then I've had five surgeries, including a full liver transplant, a broken ankle, a feeding tube, a trach, and two hernia surgeries in the past two years. So no, I can't jump like I used to. Then she had my loving husband throw a ball at me…which I'm sure he probably enjoyed too much for my liking. Then the Boss said that I may be sore the next day. Bullshit. Two days later my legs are still shaking. My skinny pants will not fit around my big old thighs and keep falling off of my nonexistent butt. You think it's funny? Go out, and jump on your kids' trampoline, and see how good you can do. No kids (congratulations)? Just stand in the middle of your floor, squat down as far as you can, and then *jump*! Just like you used to be kick-ass at volleyball or basketball.

At this point I usually run into a writer's block. Do *not* put this book down; I have plenty other things to talk about! Let's talk music. I have several different lists, for example: Exercise (obviously for workout time), Chill (for cooldown time), and Bath (for getting all the sweat off). It is important to find music that you really enjoy. For my exercise, I prefer ska bands.

Some folks don't know what ska music is. It is a form of alternative rock music mixed with bluegrass. I know it sounds confusing, but if you listen to it, you will understand. I would suggest starting light with bands such as Reel Big Fish. They have three really motivating songs: "Take On Me" (yes, I know that's a remake). Then there is "She Has a Girlfriend Now" and "Beer." I am aware that some of the language may be offensive to some, so I have some more selections to choose from. Try Smash Mouth's song "Why Can't We Be Friends?" It very motivational and upbeat. Definitely check OK Go. My favorite song and video is "Here We Go Again." Not only is it fun to work out to, the video is *awesome* to watch. I am currently listening to my personal list, and I'm having trouble not singing out loud because my husband is napping. Anyway, I will get back to my list for you guys. Definitely check out "They Might Be Giants." My all-time favorite song of theirs is "It's Istanbul, Not Constantinople." Not only is it motivational, the lyrics are pretty fun to listen to. They were popular before my time, but I really enjoy listening to Queen; I have three songs that get me moving: "Bicycle Race," "We Will Rock You," and "Fat-Bottomed Girls." Now I know that list of songs might piss off some folks, but it motivates me to work even harder. Then there is Fatboy Slim; he has a song called "The Weapon of Choice." Please bear with me; it's not as bad as it sounds. It is very fast-paced and fun to work out to. If you look up the video, you will see that Christopher Walken dances throughout the video. Also check out Cheap Trick. I'm sure that you will recognize the song "I Want You to Want Me." Have you ever heard of 311? Two songs that I find to be good warm-ups are "Amber" and "All Mixed Up." They are upbeat, but they are slow enough to warm up to. To start getting your heart pumping, listen, and think about the artist playing the song "American Woman," by Lenny Kravitz. Yeah, just looking at the picture has my iFit blowing up. Heh heh! I guess I can't let Big D read this. All the studies I have read say that you need to work in intervening stages, so take these two songs to slow down and get a drink. The first one is "Ants Marching," by Dave Matthews. The second is by a very talented blues musician named Joe Bonamassa. My favorite song to work out to is called "Ball Peen Hammer." It still falls into the cooldown section, but you will find yourself starting to speed up. Break's over; back to 311, "Beautiful Disaster" is a good start back into your workout. Go directly into Queen's "Bicycle Ride"; I don't understand all the words, and I'm pretty sure that I should be offended by it. But it makes me want to run away from it (sorry). I have a bit of a different list because after being a boss over two hundred employees and being the head chef and owner of a successful restaurant, I have some pent-up stress in my life. I tend to think I should leave that part out.

Let's go onto some more fun workout songs. I truly love the Violent Femmes; I promise I don't have a dark side. But one of my all-time favorite songs is "Blister in the Sun." I can't help but sing it out loud and practically dance. If you have any pent-up anger, this song is for you. If not, just skip over this next one: "Brain Stew," by Green Day. It is not violent by any means; it just has a very aggressive speed to it. Lighten up with some Hammer time. That's right: "You Can't Touch This." Watch the video; it will remind you of how ridiculous those pants were. Play some Dexys Midnight Runners. You don't know who they are? Think about "Come On Eileen." Your toes should be tapping now. Time to slow down for just a bit; listen to some Grouplove: "Colours." It is slower but still has a good pace. I do not like to sound creepy again, but I really like Radiohead cover of "Creep," by Macy Gray, but now that I listen to the words again, I notice there are some words that I missed. So I apologize ahead of time. Back to the motivational music. Hold onto your treadmill handles; it's time for "The Final Countdown." Now that's not an excuse to stop now, but if you need to, read ahead to the cooldown section. I always use it when I'm baking or making microwave popcorn. If you're still with me, let's dance "Gangnam Style." This may possibly be the most irritating song, but it will make my butt run trying to get through it. Let's go fun and retro: "The Golden Age," by the Asteroids Galaxy Tour. Superfun! If you are still with me, we'll walk " I'm Gonna Be" (500 Miles) with the Proclaimers. How about some "Ice Ice Baby"? Yeah, me either. I can't remember why he was such a heartthrob back in the day. OK, I was going to stop with the workout stuff, but I just realized that I left out the king, Elvis Presley! "A Little Less Conversation" and a little more action. Let's talk about "The End of the World as We Know It," by our good friends R.E.M. I will give you a dollar if you can tell me all the words in it. It's time to run: "Janie's Got a Gun." I know, I'm getting silly now. We need to talk about Steve Miller's "Joker." I had never heard that song until Dan came along. I think it's time for us to start cooling down.

"Sail," by AWOLNATION is a good place to start to cool down. It is hard but has a soothing baseline. Just try it; if you don't like it, don't bother downloading it. We will go onto Taj Mahal's "She Caught the Katy (And Left Me a Mule to Ride)." Do I know what that means? Not a clue. Then try Cake's cover of Willie Nelson's song "Sad Songs and Waltzes." Go into some sappy stuff: Jimmy Durante's "As Time Goes By." And a personal favorite is "At Last," by the great Etta James. I'm going to have to stop because I'm getting sappy. Other great songs are Johnny Cash's cover of the song "The First Time Ever I Saw Your Face" and "Wonderful Tonight," by Sir Eric Clapton. That will make everyone's heart jump a beat. The song that Dan and I chose for our first dance was Jamie Cullum's "What a Difference a Day Made." And the last one that gets to my heart is the one that describes us to a T: Jason Mraz's "I Won't Give Up." Now I am sitting here crying. Thanks, guys; now I need to go and love on my husband.

I've taken a few days off to write an ode to my sister; if she approves it, I'll write it in here. Fingers crossed! So here it goes.

Five

ODE TO DEBBY, NOT DEBBIE, ON HER BIRTHDAY

If you meet my sister, Debby, don't *dare* spell her name any different. She carries a gun and has no qualms about using it. So just mind your manners around her.

I give credit for all of the smarts, and smartassed comments, to my loving (and sometimes scary) sister. She spent day after day sitting me in front of her Apple IIe. Yes, remember, this was the early 1980s. The screen was as big as her glasses. Heh. I have no worries; she won't read this until tomorrow, so I'm safe for a few hours.

Here come the compliments. She spent all of those hours teaching me how to read and write using the Sesame Street app, or whatever they used to call it back then. Now that I think about it, I remember that it was called a "floppy disk." We played that every day, and by the time I went to kindergarten, I knew all of my letters and numbers, and I could read and write. Of course, at that point, I thought that I was the shit. Yep, I learned that from Debby, too. It got me in trouble when I was a kid—and as an adult as well.

Debby is the *only* person who has intimated me with her smarts. She took her ACTs when the top score was 40, and she got a 38. I took it when the top score was 36, and I got a 32. Then we decided to get our IQs tested; of course, she got 150, and I got a mere 149. Her only genius child outscores both myself and her mother on everything, especially when it comes to the cool factor. We'll talk about her later. She needs her own chapter, as does Debby's wonderful husband, John.

At this point it is all about Deborah Lynn. Heh, here comes another ass kicking. I got named Amanda Beth, because my mom wanted me to be Amanda Lynn but then realized that it would result in "a mandolin" (say it together really fast). So then Debby tells me that I was named for songs by Kiss and Chicago. She also told me that we had a brother in prison because he killed our real dad. His name was Junior. So as a young kid who could be easily confused, I started writing him letters. She promised she would mail them. One day I couldn't find Deb, so I took the letter to Mom and asked her to mail it. She asked me what it was, and being the naïve kid I was, I told her what it was. That's when I heard the words that I wasn't supposed to hear. I have no clue what she said to Deb. Sorry, Sis.

Let's talk sisterly music. I have pictures of sitting on her back with big-ass headphones on my head, in my pajamas, socks not matching. She had these posters of Kiss on her walls, which scared the shit out of me. But she gave me a good understanding of how good their music was. The posters still scare me, even though I've seen them without the makeup. I tend to think that is worse. Then I learned all about Prince: "Little Red Corvette," "Purple Rain," and my favorite, "Raspberry Beret."

Debby married John, whom I love with everything in me. She told me on a Tuesday that they were getting married that Thursday and made me promise not tell anyone, especially my parents. They had never met John, and to be honest, he looked like a pot-smoking hippie, which is what he was. Sorry, John. I feel like I'm having to apologize a lot right now. They worked together, and he just happened to be her mailman. I went back home, and of course, they asked how my visit went and what we talked about. I promise, it just slipped out. I said that Debby was getting married. My mom swelled up with joy, but I could see that my dad wasn't happy. He was never a happy man. At any rate, Mom was getting excited, wondering what to wear and what gifts to get them and what she was going to dress me in. She was bouncing around the house in joy, while Dad sat in his chair, being grumpy, as always.

Mom scooped me up in her excitement and asked when the wedding was. I had to bite my lip and say, "On Thursday?" Mom said, "You mean *next* Thursday, right?" Nope. Then Dad jumps up and says, "What the fuck is her last name going to be?" I had no clue, so I covered it up by saying that he was a really nice man. Well, at this point, I knew that I was in the shitter. She would never talk to me again. She did, which made me very happy.

They bought a house and completely redid it, and they invited me to come visit. I had my own room with brand-new carpet. Debby didn't realize that the fumes were very strong. She is a great cook, so she made Italian beef; it was delicious! When I was in bed, I started feeling kind of nauseous. I yelled for Deb, but before she could get in there, I rolled over and puked *all* over her brand-new carpet. Now, for sure, I've fucked up my relationship with my sister and her new husband. No, she cleaned me up, wrapped me up, and let me sleep with the best dog ever, Moose. Moose was a beautiful Great Dane, and she outweighed me by one hundred pounds. She, however, was the biggest cuddle bug ever. She just curled up to me and let me love on her all night. When it was time to get up, she would take her big, slobbery tongue and run it up my face, as if to say, "It's time to get up, sister." Every time I would come over, she would jump on me and almost knock me down. As soon as I sat down, she would be on my lap, making sure that I was being taken care of. Debby has had a few good dogs...and a few satanic dogs, too. I loved Moose, Ginger, Rosie, Spaz (yes, Spaz), Reefer, Cadbury, and Katrina—this was one of the Satan dogs. She was beautiful, but just as her namesake, Hurricane Katrina, she tore up *everything* in her path.

Back to music. Well, first, let me explain that we went different directions in life; Debby was raising Emily, working, and going to school. I was going to school, hosting parties, and bootlegging booze in from Tennessee. Anyway, we both came out OK. She became a kick-ass auditor, with her master's degree. I went school as a premed at SIU. I decided that wasn't for me, so I went to Murray State and graduated with a bachelor's in social services.

In all of this, I married Dan, and I worked my way through the group-home system from a direct care worker to the director. I did this for nine years, so Dan told me to go back to school. I went and got my culinary degree, became the best chef in town, and even owned a very popular Italian restaurant.

What does this have to do with me and my sister? I just wanted to explain why we were apart so long. There were no bad feelings; we were both busy.

So we finally got back together and started hanging out. We went to Jamaica, Memphis, Chicago, and Wisconsin. Emily was a big WWE fan, so we took her to a match and made her a big neon sign, and it was so big, you could see her on TV. Then Deb and I got the great idea to go to a Korn concert. Of course, we wanted to get close to the front, so the couple we went with—a good friend of mine and her *very* large but sweet husband—came with us. Of course, you have to drink a couple of beers before the concert. We were superexcited because we had front-row seats. However, when we got there, they had oversold the tickets. That meant it was standing room only. We worked our way to the front. Everyone was lined up just fine. As soon as the lights went out and the band came out, we started smelling weed. That's when it turned into a huge mosh pit. Remember, Deb wears huge glasses. We were getting pushed around. I was fine; I'm tall and sturdy. Debby started getting pushed around, and someone pushed her and jammed her big-ass glasses into her eye, blackening it. I found the fucker who pushed her, and I started pushing the living shit out of him. I was winning, and I started to throw punches, but then I was grabbed from behind. A tall, scary African-American gentleman who came up, grabbed the guy who was pushing us around by the throat, and "took care of him." I have no idea what happened to him, but we all came out OK.

I had my own apartment at this time, so they got me settled in. At this point I was just messaging Big D online.

Debby, John, Emily (who calls me "Mandy" and Dan "Unkie Dan"), Daniel (he hates it when I call him that, but he will learn), and I eventually did.

So with all of this, happy belated birthday, Debbie! (I mean Debby. Heh, heh.)

Six

Friends and Family

It has been a while since I've written. So I decided to go in a different direction altogether. Let's talk about good times with friends and family. I've already talked about my family. There is my genius and smartassed sister and my lovable brother-in-law, John. There is my supersmart niece, Emily. Finally, there is my mom, Daphine (Momma D), whom no one will play games with—why? Because she *cheats* at every game; she has earned the title "Dirty Poker [or Rummy] Cheater." She uses the fact she has early onset Alzheimer's disease. I think she just cheats, as does everyone in the family.

Dan's family is complicated. Don't get me wrong; I love them all very much. Mom and Dad are awesome. His brother and sister-in-law have a very beautiful baby girl. I really feel bad for her; she is currently teething. I'm glad I can't remember that point in my life.

My friends are spread far and away. Most of my best friends live close. There are Jamie and Anita, who visited me in the hospital all the time. Also Tim and Amy, Darby, and Christy were constantly in my room. I feel bad because they remember visiting me, but I have no recollection of them ever being there. I was especially ashamed that I couldn't remember Christy's name; I just called her "Darby's wife." They are all very close, but my long-distance best friends are too far away.

My best hillbilly friend, Sara, and I cause so much trouble. I would love to tell you about them, but they may have been illegal. Shh. But we did have so much fun in haunted houses. She nearly choked me when we went to a really scary house. I was wearing a hoodie, and she was walking behind me. Something jumped out at her; she got scared and pulled on my hoodie. Good times. Then there is Jessica, whom you will talk to if you are having customer problems. She is married to a *very* successful heart physician's assistant. He does vital surgeries on people with heart issues. I can't forget Bruce—great guy, but he lives in Indy. He is a nursing instructor at one of the many hospitals.

I can't leave out Frank and Gina, the power couple from whom bought my restaurant. I sincerely love both of them and their kids. Gina is the model of a smart, beautiful business executive. I am sure she has the patience of a saint. OK, maybe I am kissing up a bit; she makes it easy to look up to her. Now, Frank is a different story. We had an instant connection for two reasons. First, he was willing to take the time to teach me. I think the only reason I got hired was because he needed free labor (I was an intern for school). I had a pretty impressive résumé. I was about to graduate from culinary school, and I had been a social worker for the previous nine years. My first initiation to the store was to see how many times I could run up and down the poorly lit and very steep steps to grab supplies that we needed. On a busy day, that could be three to four times a shift. Second, my initiation was to see how many times I could be called "Amanda Hug and Kiss." If you don't know that reference, it comes from *The Simpsons*.

Shortly after that I "got" to run the cash register. At that point, I was able to take food to the tables without dropping it. He then asked me into the kitchen and let me do whatever I wanted. What's cool about the restaurant was that we just cooked or made the sandwiches that we thought the customers would like that day. We carried only the best meats (both domestic and foreign). The same was with the cheeses. This made us an exclusive destination. We got our liquor licenses for beer and wine. Frank knew everything about wine. We had some really good wine reps. Dan, at that point, was becoming a beer connoisseur. He was able to give Frank good advice to get the very best beer. We got our licenses so we could serve in-house wine and beer. Tim, my best friend, came and built a very contemporary stainless-steel bar. Frank painted the walls a burnt orange. We then set the tables so everyone could bask in the sunshine and view our perfect view of the Ohio River.

By this time we were getting really busy. Frank, Jess, and I were busting our asses to put out the best food in the tri-state area. Anna and Andrea *ran* the desk like real champs. We had a great pastry chef. We could give her any goofy request, and she could knock it out. At this point, Frank asked me to purchase the store, and I was proud to say *yes*! We ran it for two and a half very successful years. We were doing in-house dinners, grab-and-go dinners, wine and beer tastings… it was amazing! It did, however, begin to get overwhelming, and I was starting to get sick.

Dan and I had to sell the store when I got sick, so now I sit and write this book. I still talk to Francis (he hates being called that). He is still my friend, and I still look up to him for advice. I even have a bobblehead of him. When I get upset regarding the closing of the business, I will walk by his bobblehead and thunk him on his head to say, "Thanks, Frank, for getting me into this mess." He had no idea what I was going to have to go through. Oh, well. Who's to blame?

In fact, I talked to him this morning. Apparently I am not the only one who has unreasonable dreams about our store. I say "our store" because he and I were opening a store with only our business sense and our culinary knowledge. I went to culinary school; he traveled the world, experiencing all each country had to offer. We were the power team of small-town Indiana.

Apparently, talking to him reminded me of some of my best recipes.

Bacon Jam

This is one of my favorites. I am well known as being a lover of all things pork. Then, I got to thinking about ways to put it in everything I could eat throughout the day…*bacon jam*!

It's way easy to make. I used to make a sandwich with it (turkey BLT with bacon jam). Not only was it tasty, but it made for a great picture. Bacon jam is the perfect blend of salty and sweet, but it can be used as a condiment or as a dessert accompaniment. You will need the following ingredients:

- 1 lb. bacon (diced)
- 1 large onion (diced)
- 4 large cloves garlic (minced)
- 1 tsp. crushed red pepper (or to taste)
- ½ tsp. cracked black pepper
- 1 Tbsp. cumin
- 2 tsp. mustard
- 4 oz. bourbon (I suggest you get a good one), the kind that you would have over a couple of cubes of ice
- 1 Tbsp. apple cider vinegar
- Salt to taste

Sauté bacon over medium/high heat for 5 minutes (until bacon has just started to brown). Reduce the temp; add onion. Sauté for 5 more minutes until it becomes translucent. Add garlic. Sauté 2 minutes.

Add black pepper, red pepper, cumin, and mustard; stir. Remove from heat, and then add bourbon. Return to low heat, and let simmer until the meat and veggies are completely soft. Let cool, and at this point, taste for seasoning, especially for salt. Pulse in a food processor 4–5 minutes until jam is spreadable. Enjoy as a condiment, a sandwich spread, or as a dessert ingredient. I would suggest spreading it on a toasted baguette and then adding a sharp cheese like Brie or taleggio.

The following recipe was developed by my pastry chef.

<u>Bagel bombs with goat (or any kind of) cheese, bacon, and scallions</u>
This is a spin on the traditional bagel. In this case, the toppings are baked inside the bagels. Crazy, right? *Yes!* In the best possible way. I prefer goat cheese, but I know that some folks don't care for goat cheese. Plan on making the dough quite a bit before you want serve the bagels. They will have to need to rise for 45 minutes. I would suggest that you start that first. First, gather all of your ingredients.

For the filling:

- 3½ oz. bacon
- 1.4 oz. goat cheese, or cream cheese if you prefer
- 1 bunch of scallions, thinly sliced
- 2 tsp. sugar
- 1 tsp. kosher salt

For the mother dough:

- 3½ cups flour
- 1 Tbsp. kosher salt
- 1⅛ tsp active dry yeast
- 1¾ water, room temp
- 1 tsp. veggie oil

For the egg wash and poppy-seed topping:

- 1 egg at room temp
- ½ cup water at room temp
- 4 tsp. poppy seeds
- ¾ tsp. kosher salt
- ½ tsp. onion powder
- ¼ tsp. garlic powder
- Sesame seeds
- Punch dough down, and flatten the dough on a smooth, dry countertop. Use a dough cutter to cut into 16 equal parts. Use your fingers to gently stretch each piece of dough into a flat circle.
- Put a frozen ball of cream cheese (with the bacon and scallions inside) in the center plug until completely contained. Roll the ball between your hands to make a perfect ball, to ensure that it is a nice round shape.
- Spread the bombs with egg wash, and then top generously with your poppy-seed mixture.
- Arrange the bombs 4 inches apart on either a Silpat or a parchment paper–lined baking pan.
- Bake for 20–30 minutes at 325° F. While in the oven, the bombs will become a deep golden brown, and a few may have explosions. If you are brave enough, you can tuck the cheese back in. When they are ready, serve immediately!

Seven

MY MOM PICKED A PICKLED
PECK OF PETER PEPPERS

Apparently this chapter is about Momma D. It starts with me drinking a big cup of milk. My sister and I made a beautiful salad. I was *so* excited that I had found a jar of my mom's famous "pickled peppers," so I decided to put them on my salad. *Bad* mistake! It lit up my tongue—and my ass! I then listened to all the angry music I had in my playlist. At that point I decided to call Momma D and tell her exactly what had happened. Did she apologize? Nope. She said, "I can only imagine what it is going to feel like coming out." Really? I guess I should have expected this from the same woman who, when I got struck with lightning and had the wind knocked out of me, nudged me with her foot, leaned over me, and said, "You best start breathing." Who says that to a barely breathing child? My mom says that! To top it off, the lightning hit my Great Dane, Babe, at the exact same time. So then Momma D had a Great Dane and her child cuddled up on the couch together because we were both scared to death! She really is a good mom; she can't cook, but she is a love bug. For that reason I went to culinary school, as did my niece, Emily. My sister has always been a good cook. Now we feed Mom because she doesn't have to cook anymore.

Some of my favorite memories are from going to the Kentucky Derby. We had so much fun picking out our *big* hats and pretty floral dresses. We went to the best Cuban restaurant we have ever been to. She immediately fell in love with the coffee, so much so that she had three cups of it. We didn't have the heart to tell her that it was turbocharged. That made for a *long* ride home! That was probably one of the best times she and I had in a long time…other than when my cousins and I got drunk, took her to the bar, and had her order a drink (she is not a drinker). Then we took her to the porn store and did everything that we could to embarrass the shit out of her. Good times. I'm not brave enough to take my mom-in-law there yet; she still thinks that I am a good kid.

Eight

I'm Finally Learning about Who I Am

It's only taken me thirty-six years, a ton of physical and mental challenges, and good people pushing me around. You know, I have stepped away from this book for a couple of weeks because I ran out of ideas, but now that I'm back…that sentence really pisses me off. Not one person has *pushed* me to do anything. I just realized that I am the one pushing myself too damn hard. I complain about being sore, but then I have to tell myself, "I am sore because I'm working so hard to get better." Just over a year ago, I could not walk, talk, or eat without twenty-four-hour care. Who the hell am I to complain?

So I have decided to stop complaining (unless it genuinely hurts) and suck it up, put a shit-eating grin on my face, and just do it. I am constantly telling people, "Suck it up, buttercup." I guess I should start following my own advice, huh? I have sat down and made out a list of things I want to accomplish over the next few months. This has really motivated me to start working harder. It would be my suggestion that you do the same thing.

I just had a benefit thrown for me by my good friends. I was surprised to see how many people came out to support me! It was a truly humbling experience! They raised nearly $3,500. I couldn't express my thanks enough. I ended up buying a purse that I later found out my sister had donated. If I had known, I would have asked her for it!

On a different note, I just had to get three teeth surgically removed earlier this week. It felt great when they numbed me, but it began to suck shortly after that. I am a bit concerned because I have speech therapy today; I hope she will be forgiving, as I have to keep gauze in my mouth all the time now. When I'm not feeling well, I speak very quietly, believe it or not. Wish me luck! All I want is "sick soup" and my sister's secret recipe for "sick tea" as well. I know the recipes for both, but it is not the same if I have to make it myself.

So I guess it is time for me to get back to me bettering myself. I'm currently working with my local vocational rehabilitation office. They are willing to get me driving lessons and a part-time job, either working as a job coach, which I had done for several years, or teaching people with disabilities how to cook. This is something that I am interested in doing anyway! If you have a disability, it is normal to want to shake someone silly! So many times, I have worked with folks who may have physical disabilities but are geniuses who can't express their smarts! It is so frustrating to me because I have seen it time and time again. People need to understand that it may take some time for folks to gather up either the courage or their thoughts before they are willing to share them with us. Maybe we *all* should take that lesson ourselves! Even I have that problem. I scored some of the highest possible scores on my standardized tests. I got into Ivy League schools; however, I get looked down upon because I have a brain injury. I limp, and sometimes my speech gets slurred, especially when I am tired. So shut it! Think about your words before you speak! I have a cousin who is a savant but can't express himself. He worked his way through a junior college and then began to write political speeches for local senators and representatives—even one gentleman who was running for president! I have always been protective of him because some of his siblings would tell him that he was stupid. No! He was far from stupid; he just didn't have the ability to "speak" his thoughts. He just needed the opportunity to write them out! So again, check yourself before you judge someone. You never know who is judging you.

Nine

Perhaps I Need to Put Some Happy Music On?

I tend to get frustrated when I see people being judged, especially if they have disabilities. It seems today that you can be judged by *anything* now. I refuse to get into political discussions anymore. I can't even watch the news! I need to take that back; I'm addicted to watching YouTube videos on Facebook. I happened to run across one video that talked about the Paralympics. That is amazing to see! The gentleman narrating the video said that this year, there were more Olympic records broken during these games, including bicycle speed racing. The four-hundred-meter men's relay was a group of gentlemen who had sight deficiencies. Even with these, they broke records. There is a picture on the site of them holding their gold medals. My husband gets mad at me when I say that I have a disability. He thinks that I'm giving in to it, but on the contrary, I'm embracing it so that I can prove my recovery mostly to myself, but also those naysayers who say there is no recovery for ODS. It is true that most of us die young, but there are many of us who have worked our asses off to better ourselves and the people around us!

So if you are reading this and have a disability, here is my advice: "Suck it up, buttercup." Please don't be offended, but I had to tell myself that every time I fell down or got hurt from working out. It truly works! Over the years I have worked with many people with different abilities. (At this point, I feel like I should be saying "different abilities.") Every one of us has different quirks. Saying this, we all have our setbacks, too. I confess that I will drink a cup of coffee, add two shots of espresso, and then wash it down with a Red Bull. Then an hour later, I am complaining about the terrible headache I have. Can I blame that on my disability? Nope! That, my friends, is one person with OCD and a Type A personality, who refuses to stop until it is all finished. Whew! That makes me tired just thinking about it.

Let's talk happy stuff. I've not been typing much lately because so much good has been going on! Last week I walked a 5K. Well, I walked half of it and then went to the huge grocery and walked the rest of it. It was 3.33 miles, to be exact! Dan and I got a new puppy. Her name is LuLu. She is an English springer spaniel, and she fits all the characteristics of the breed. She is supersmart, very fast, and very stubborn and feisty. She has decided that our shoes, socks, underwear, wood furniture, and fingers are all her personal chew toys. I've been calling D and me her pork chops.

I also went to vocational rehabilitation yesterday. We had to make the trip up to Indy again. The people were very nice; however, they put me through six hours of testing. With only one break, my brain was exhausted! Dan and I first met with the neuropsychologist, who explained all the testing that I would have to endure. Testing began simply with general orientation: place, time, year, date, past and present presidents, and so on. Then there were different memory tasks:

drawing, reading, writing, math, vision testing, and reaction timing. The second part consisted of personal questions and then vocational questions. Needless to say, I slept well that night.

I've decided that I would like to teach people with autism how to cook. I spent nine years specializing in autism behavioral disorders. I feel like after two years of culinary school and two and a half years of owning a restaurant, I can teach these folks. Everyone deserves the right to learn whatever he or she wants to. I want to teach these folks!

As I've been talking about myself, I have noticed some things that have changed since my brain injury. Apparently several other people have as well. That being said, I was given a list of things to think about before acting on my first thought. Think about this for yourself.

- What overstimulates you or easily distracts you?
- How do you feel physically and mentally when getting overstimulated?
- What happens when overstimulated emotionally, verbally, or when interacting with others?

I thought this would be a good idea as this is due in a couple of days. Yes, when you get good therapists, you get homework…just like school.

Ten

I'm Starting to See the Bright Side

I just realized that in January 2017, I will have been on this journey for three whole years. I will also be turning thirty-seven, which I hate to admit. But I am finally getting my memory back, long and short, which has been tough for me. People don't believe that I could hear everything that was said while I was in a coma. Especially music. It took me three weeks to wake up. That's when I had no recollection of any time, days, or my location. It was frustrating, because I didn't recognize my family and friends.

As time goes by, things start to come back. I've seen photos of me when I was very sick, skinny, and practically orange. It jogged my memory of how terrible dialysis was. But on the bright side, I made friends with many of the patients and nurses. Mind you, the side effects were terrible, but it got me ready for the transplant. The transplant was life-changing, and yes, I had many issues, including a brain injury. It was a life-changing event; however, I am, happily, alive. I just found out my donor was a seventeen-year-old male. This young man saved five lives with his liver, two kidneys, corneas, and bone marrow.

What an amazing young man! There is no way to contact his family. There is a part me of that wants to say "Thank you," but I'm afraid it would be too hard on me and the family. So, family, if you ever read this book—thank you.

Now I can remember all of my childhood, which my mom isn't thrilled with. Everyone is more concerned with my short-term memory. Here is my suggestion to work on that. You might not like this, but it is my favorite thing to do. *Make lists!* And put them in places where you will find them. No cheating! My suggestion is to purchase a dry-erase calendar and hang it somewhere you will always see it.

My calendar lives on my refrigerator (my favorite spot in the house). I change it each month. Dates are always in black. Doctor appointments are in green. Therapy appointments are in blue. For personal appointments I coordinate the color by event. I write my goals down the side. My goals for this month are:

- Work on book
- Plan menus for four days
- Help with training LuLu
- Pay more attention to Booker
- Keep up with laundry, dishes, floors, and the closet

This seems like a huge list, and it is, but I *will* complete it before the end of the month! Mark off goals as you meet them. It will start building your confidence. It helps me to focus, which is a problem for me. It gradually builds my faith in myself and my newfound abilities. In the past year and a half, I have learned to walk, talk, speak, and eat. I walked the 5K for my community physical therapy group. I've started to teach cooking classes. I'm obviously writing a book. Do these need to be your accomplishments? No! Start slow, with simple goals, then build, and build, and build until you are starting to reaching your goals. When you do that, make bigger goals. Keep your head up. "Suck it up, buttercup!" There is no doubt in my mind that you and I can beat our setbacks.

You know, I don't know what gets you down or discourages you. Here is a good idea. Everyone knows that I throw my own pity party, but I decided to throw a party for my friends and family. My all-time favorite Halloween! Dan and I cooked enough food for an army. Fifteen of our good friends and family came in costume. We ate, drank, ate more, and spent some time around our fire pit. We ate all the trick-or-treat candy. Thank goodness, we only had enough for the trick-or-treaters. Oops!

Here are my goals for the next year:

- Relearn how to drive
- Walk another 5K
- Finish this book
- Completely clean my house
- Go back to work
- Start to professionally teach people with disabilities how to cook

Do you know what your goals are? Go somewhere quiet, put some music on, and take some snacks (you always need snacks for good thinking). Get a pen and paper or a journal, and write down answers to the following questions:

- What is bothering you?
- Why?
- What steps do you need take to make this better?

Now the good stuff (start snacking):

- What do I want to do tomorrow?
- How about the rest of the week?
- Can I make a plan for the week?
- Can I write out a monthly calendar?
- What goals can I accomplish this month?
- *Write them down!*
- Go get some more snacks, and just think it over.

Don't be embarrassed by your goals. They are distinctly yours. I encourage you to embrace them and be proud of them! Of course you will have naysayers. Show them up! You are better than that. These are your goals!

No, I am not getting on to you. I just want to encourage you to stand up for yourself. If you're anything like me, you internalize the bad things, and it seems like you can't get past them. That is bullshit. If you have had to fight to regain some skills, you can fight the bad stuff. I'm not saying go out with fury—think it through! It is amazing how having a calm approach can make you feel more positive. I know, I know—every self-help book says this; however, those authors have educators who have studied this for years. Yes, those are helpful, but they haven't been in your shoes.

I haven't walked in *your* shoes, but I have walked in a pretty shitty pair of shoes. It is not my sob story. It is meant to be inspirational. I do have an education in social services. I spent nine years advocating for people with physical and intellectual disabilities. It gave me a true perspective into what they experience, not being to express their feelings. In my past journey, I have been in their shoes, too—not being able to walk, talk, speak, or even breathe on my own. I now understand why they would lash out when trying to communicate and not able to get their thoughts out. It resulted in head banging, biting, or lashing out at staff. You may understand, but if you do not, please think about it.

Eleven

If You Like Cooking Comfort Food, Read On

I know that I harp on cooking, but it can either be relaxing or maddening. Start slow and simple. Dan's mom, Janice, told him, "If you can cook ground beef, you can make anything you need to live on." Dan took that to heart. On our second date, he showed up with a Crock-Pot, ground beef, and a chili mix. Was it good? Nope. For the past twelve years, I have been making the chili—or trying to teach him how to do it.

Ground beef is a magical ingredient. A person can make burgers. Who doesn't love burgers? Do not be afraid to buy mixes like Hamburger Helper, Manwich, or spaghetti sauce. There is no shame in that. Be adventurous; make meatloaf, tacos, or meatballs. Again, don't be afraid of ramen noodles; make them with chicken broth, and add some hot sauce. You cannot beat that for $1.00 for ten packets. When you get comfortable, add some chives, garlic powder, or minced onions. Hey! Make macaroni and cheese. You can do *anything* with mac and cheese. Add broccoli, chicken, leftover chili; some people like tomatoes and hot sauce. Add some chicken, rice, and broccoli; put it in a greased pan, bake it at 350° F for 25 minutes (if the chicken is already cooked), top it with cheese, and voilà—you have a casserole! Some people like to do it with tuna, ham, different veggies, tofu, eggs, or any other type of meat.

Eggs are your friend. Scramble at first; then, hard-boil them. Here's a tip. Boil them for ten minutes, and then turn off the heat, and let them rest in the hot water for five minutes. Carefully transfer the eggs to a bath of cold water with ice in it. Let them sit until completely cold, and they will be easier to peel. Only peel them as you eat them; store the rest in the fridge to keep them fresh. Once you get comfortable with the eggs, start frying them, and try to make an omelet (don't be discouraged; they never come out right the first few times). Invest in an egg poacher; it will take the stress out of manually doing it.

One can't forget the humble potato. What can't you do to a potato? You can mash it. Bake it. Hell, if you are mad enough at it, bake it again! This time, be sure to add butter, cheese, bacon, sour cream, and chives. If you are supermad at it, put some screaming hot chili and hot sauce on it. That will show that potato. Honestly, you can use potatoes for many dishes. French fries come to my mind. Just promise you will not buy them at a fast-food restaurant. You can do it healthier at home and make them taste even better. You have three choices:

- Fry, which is messy and will stink up your house.
- Bake, which takes patience but can be a creative method.
- Or you can grill or smoke your potatoes, which will give you a unique flavor.

How should you do these?

Fry

- Decide if you like skins on or off. Once you choose, wash, peel (or not), and *dry*—you don't want splattering!
- If you have a deep fryer, add veggie oil to the line, turn it to 305° F, and gently lower the basket into the fryer.
- Cook for 3–5 minutes, watching for color change.
- Pull when desired, and drain on paper towels.
- Season with salt and pepper, seasoned salt, garlic powder, hot sauce, cumin, lime…whatever you like.
- If you do not have a deep fryer, find a deep pan you can fry in.
- Follow the same directions as above.

Bake

- Now, you can do this with regular potatoes or sweet potatoes.
- When baking, I always suggest leaving the skins on. Why? That is where the nutrients and flavor come from.
- *Make sure you wash the hell out of them!* Potatoes grow underground, and you don't want to expose anyone to whatever is under there!
- I like to wrap mine in foil, poke a few holes in the foil, and roast them at 350° F for at least 30–45 minutes.
- Unwrap one, and test it with a fork; if almost done, take the potatoes out of the oven, and leave them wrapped for carryover cooking. Carryover cooking is when food continues to cook after being removed from the heat source.
- If it is complete to your liking, you can serve with condiments as guests would like them. Turn your kitchen into a potato bar. Offer butter, sour cream, cheese, bacon, and chives.

- Now, if you need a kicked-up potato, like me, put it in an ovenproof dish, and load the hell out of it. Bake or broil it for 2–4 minutes.
- Or kill it with some chili!
- You can do the same with sweet potatoes, too. Open one up; put in an ovenproof dish; and load it with butter, marshmallows, brown sugar, cinnamon, and, if you're brave enough, some cayenne, too. Good luck (heh heh)!

Grilling and smoking
Grilling:

- Cut the potatoes into ½-inch-thick slices lengthwise.
- Place them, side by side, on a sheet of aluminum foil that you have lined with bacon.
  Drizzle the potatoes with veggie oil; I also like rosemary, garlic, salt, and pepper.
- Close the foil, and grill over moderate heat until you smell the bacon.
- Check, and make sure the bacon is cooked.
- Let it rest and carryover.
- Serve with a tasty steak!

Smoking:

- My favorite!
- Still keep the skins on. This is easy!
- Build a fire with a gentle fruit wood—apple, peach, or cherry.
- After washing the taters, wrap them in foil.
- Add butter or veggie oil, salt and pepper, and some hard herbs, if you like.

- Poke holes in the foil, and place the potatoes on the smoker.
- Maintain a temp of 250° F for 30–45 minutes, depending on how many you are cooking.
- I recommended serving with smoked beef ribs or pulled-pork sandwiches.

So, beginner to pro, you have the skills to live. Don't be afraid to buy quality lunch meat (Boar's Head is my favorite, by far). Use the skills you have learned to make kick-ass sandwiches! Invest in a panini press, and experiment. Heck, start with a fancy grilled cheese! Find some smoked Gouda, fresh mozzarella, sharp Swiss, Havarti, Brie—anything other than American slices! Just butter the outsides of your bread, add cheese, put the other piece on, and impress everyone—especially if you serve it with soup, salad, and a good glass of crisp white wine.

One can also buy a great meal. It doesn't have to be simple. Splurge on some thin crackers, cream cheese, and smoked salmon, and grab some capers and lemon juice! You can eat all day on that. Invest in a few "fancy" ingredients—things like sundried tomatoes, capers, artichoke hearts, Greek olives, and some good, crispy bread. You can make appetizers and a damn good pizza. Get some veggies on sale and some hummus, and you have a great snack. Mix it with some rice and a pita, and you have a meal. If you need protein and don't want to cook, grab some tofu or a precooked chicken. If I'm feeling short on protein, I grab some protein drinks when they are on sale. They can be expensive, but you can find them 10 for $10 at some stores. You just have to watch the ads. String cheese is good protein; so is my favorite, yogurt, and I add fruit to it. It is easy to get pulled in by commercials for those "protein snacks," which end up being string cheese wrapped in lunch meat; you can do that at home if you invest in some sandwich baggies to keep them fresh. If you plan ahead, you can buy this one time, and it will last you to your next shopping trip. It's all about planning!

Twelve

Relearning How to Deal with Disappointment

No, this is not a downer chapter, but I've come to realize some things about myself that I was trying to avoid—things that I already knew. Last month I had to go to Indianapolis for some cognitive testing. I was disappointed to find that my IQ was only 87. The testers also told me that I only had a reading level of a twelfth grader. I saw red, because I graduated college with a degree and then went on to culinary school. It took three people telling me not to fret because this is just a picture of "right now." That makes sense now, but at the time, I was ready to kick some ass. Six months ago I could not have even taken the test. Six months from now, I will ace the tests. I've come to realize that healing is a process. Unfortunately, it cannot be rushed. Damn it! You may not have a brain injury, like me, but you might have some cognitive issues as well. So what? You have to heal, too! It might take therapy or just a good support system. Either way, you have to find the drive within yourself to get back to your old self…or even better!

- Get out of the house.
- Give someone a hug.
- Put on some workout clothes, and go for a walk.
- Come home, and shower.
- Put on some jammies, and cuddle up to hot coffee and a book, or a beer and a game.
- Don't feel guilty; you just worked out.
- Realize that you can't be "on" all the time. It's OK to take a time-out.

I've realized that when life kicks you in the ass, you buck up and kick it right back! You know, I wish I had thought about that a *long* time ago, like chapters back. It has taken me 26,560 words to come up with that shit! Sorry about that. You've had to read this all the way to get to the point. This shit gets better! When I was thinking about the title, I was just starting to think about how maybe hearing how bad I've had it will inspire people.

I have almost died twice. I've had tubes in every orifice. I'm grateful to have a liver donor who saved my life. I am a thankful woman— more thankful than I can ever put on pages. Please do not think that I am not. In that same breath, I'm tired of feeling sorry for myself. Do I hurt every day? Yes! Do I still complain about it? Yes! Why? I thought it was because I was weak—but no, I'm not weak. That is the pain that comes with getting better. I still get frustrated with my inability to focus. Maybe it is because I don't take the time to think about it. It is ludicrous to blame my therapists for working me too hard. That is their damn job. I am just playing a blame game so I don't have to take the responsibility for my own care. That is bullshit, Amanda! Yes, I talk to myself when life hits me in the head. Why did I name a book *The Best Is Yet to Come* if I didn't know if it would be coming? Beats me. Maybe wishful thinking? It was eight months ago when I started this book. I was hoping that it would get better. Lately, however, I realized that it is in *my* control. It gets better when I decide it will.

Nothing will change until I change it. That means getting up on days when I don't have therapy and walking anyway, and doing my stretches on the floor every day. I work my core, arms, and wrists. I also do mind puzzles to keep my brain going. Does it get better? Yes, but it is slower than we want, or, I should say, "slower than I want." That is the case.

So here is an example of how I know I'm getting better. Today, I'm going to help some Girl Scouts make Christmas cookies for their families. I'm honored that they asked me because I'm a "professional chef," and they think that is cool. I do enjoy them, but they scare the shit out of me. More often than not, my group-home kids wanted to bite or throw things at me. I'm sure these girls won't, but girls in a group are dangerous. I take that back—maybe it was just my group. We were a competitive group who were determined to win. These girls are just getting together to make cookies. In my head, they are sweet and innocent, but I'm a girl, too. I have that behind-the-back-eye-roll thing, too.

Why talk about this? It is showing progress. I have learned to recognize something that overstimulates me, and now I can plan for it. This is a strategy that was taught to me by my speech therapist, Beth. She encouraged me to make a chart so I can keep track of what causes me unnecessary stress. This works! Try it. I keep saying to bust your ass at every aspect of your life, and it will improve. Does it suck? Yep, it does. At this, you need to take a long look in the mirror and assess yourself. Do *not* just look at flaws; we all have them. See the person you are and the person you want to be. That is when you get a plan in place and make that makes these two images come together. Take time!

So, prior to my transplant, I went to the hospital for stress tests and wasn't feeling well. They tried to set a feeding tube—to no avail.

This was from the large amount of ammonia called hepatic encephalopathy. I named it "Snuffleupagus." It felt like a big, hairy elephant on my chest and the rest of my body. I got on the list, and four days later, I got my new, shiny liver. After surgery I went to the TICU (transplant intensive care unit) where I spent over thirty days. When I had made some progress, I was sent to the OTU (organ transplant unit). This is where I met my saviors.

I had a big scare and victory all at one time. I had to go to Indy for my annual checkup. All was good—whew! When the appointment was over, we went up to the OTU, and it was a mix of emotions. It was so good to see the team: Britton, Lindy, Alisa, Taina, Carly, Mary, Amy, Christine, and Danielle. Then, the bad memories started. I could not move my neck, arms, legs, fingers, and toes. I was completely paralyzed. They told me they had to put me in a lift to move me. Shortly after arriving, I went into a coma. Terrible, right? Yep, I was there. So were they. Bad times. But there were good times, too. They had to put a tracker on me because I used to like to go *all* over the place. I even tried to break out! When I woke up, I was angry. The first words out of my mouth were "*No!*" and "Get the fuck out!" Not my best days, but they held my hands and feet and put those "squeeze things" on my legs. And I got woken up every two hours to be turned and to have my vitals and bloodwork done. They still loved on me and made me feel like family.

Have you ever read *Oh, the Places You'll Go!*, by Dr. Seuss? Of course, you have. I found my copy, reread it, and thought to myself, *Holy shit.* I totally should have read that again before I started this project. I was happy to find it. My best friend at the time had bought it for me for college. I guess she knew I was going to be the one with four different majors. I was that kid who went in for premed, engineer, social worker, and chef classes. I have enough credits to have a master's degree. I'm just glad it was on scholarships.

Back to our struggle to get better. There was a dear man in my life who has since passed. He was a wonderful man. His name was Don. He came into my deli every day and fixed himself coffee and sat at "his" table to hold court. He knew everyone, and they knew him. He was my confidant and giver of advice. Well, while reading my book, I found a quote that always warms my heart. He wrote, "Those who go slow, go far and safe." How wise? Now, I think about that with every decision I make. I suggest you do, too.

During the healing of your body and mind, you need to slow down. If you are anything like me, I think, *The harder and faster I work, the faster I will get better*. Bullshit! I end up sore and grouchy for days afterward. In my head, I'm completely healed...but I'm not. I worry all the time about my progress and if I'm living up to everyone else's standards for me. I need to slow down and walk (not run) farther and safer.

So many therapists have helped me to suck it up. Meghan is my physical therapy "Boss." Five times up and down from the floor. My dumb ass says, "Why don't I do the Superman?" This is where you lie on your stomach and put your hands and legs up in the air and act like you are flying. I'm such a stupid ass. Exercises involve stepping around canes in alternating directions, wall squats, sit-to-stands, the treadmill with ankle weights—whew!

My occupational therapist is Shannon: "Sit up straight, sister." She works on my left arm and hand. It is what bothers me the most due to my brain injury. She also helps me with my posture, obviously, as well how that affects my vision. Along with Boss, they work on my stamina, mentally and especially physically. If I have to pick one more tiny pin and put in a tiny hole, I will scream. Now that I think about it, that is just like playing golf. You chase a little ball until you get into a tiny hole 350 yards away. At least that is fun. This benefits me, but it's not fun. In the beginning, I had to wear an eye patch. My vision was so bad, that was her only way to help me correct it. I still have mine. I'm just waiting on the next Halloween!

"Concentrate" Beth is a saint. She is the one who has to put everything together and make it easy to comprehend. In the beginning I did not have a voice. After weeks of saying "Ahh" over and over, I finally got a voice. I'm sure everyone is grateful now. After many sessions of memory games, flash cards, and higher-thinking tasks, I've learned how to manage my thoughts. At one point just trying to organize cards into categories was too difficult and made me mad easily. Now it is a very simple task. I won't tell her, but it is fun.

With their help, I can do cooking classes, a future goal of mine. I told you, the best is still coming. I spend one Sunday a month with the Girl Scouts. So far we have done dips and Christmas cookies. Now tomorrow, December 11, we will be doing a brunch for the Ronald McDonald House. I am very excited. I'm thinking maybe a cinnamon-raisin focaccia. Well, I didn't have time. Good intentions.

Well, we did the brunch. It was amazing! I had never been through a Ronald McDonald House. It was amazing! The gentleman volunteer gave us a tour of two floors and the basement. Everything (mostly) is donated. While we were there, five families were staying there. If you don't know about the house, it is a house for families who have children who are sick. They can get shelter, food, and calm surroundings to find some solace. The "staff" are mostly volunteers. Small groups come in and help cook and clean to help out the families. Everyone needs to educate him- or herself and donate money or just a little bit of time to these folks. I only wish Dan had had a place like that while I was so sick. He had to sleep in a hotel or on a couch or chair in my room with me. I feel like it was as hard on him as it was on me. I was living on food pumped into me through a tube, and he was living on Payday bars and Mountain Dew. The nurses adopted him and would let him eat with them and even call in orders so he could eat with them. Our extended family. I don't think they even know it.

Thirteen

Am I ready? Nope! Since I am not employed, money is tight. This year I will be making many of the gifts. Cookies, bacon jam, candy, fruitcake, and cocoa-mix jars. I figure that it is not about how much money you spend, but that you thought to make a gift for someone. It usually means more to them anyway. When Christmas comes, so does the New Year. Hmph! I choose not to do resolutions because I am doomed to break them.

I came up with a list to accomplish this year:

- Walk on the treadmill four days a week, including PT sessions
- Plan menus four days a week in hopes of budgeting money better
- Work on losing weight and gaining muscle
- Finish and get this book published
- Work on finding a job
- Try to find a job teaching people with disabilities how to cook
- Get a driving evaluation and relearn how to drive

- Make more "date time" with Dan. You lose the time to date when you have been married for twelve years.

Countdown: Nine days to Christmas. Am I done shopping? Nope! Have I started? Nope! Will I shop? Nope, I've decided to save money and make my gifts. I spent all day yesterday with the in-laws, making bacon jam, peanut butter balls, mix-filled ornaments, cocoa-mix jars, and chocolate spoons and pretzels to go with the cocoa.

I think I'm going to try my hand at fruitcake. I've never done it, so wish me luck. My mom, Momma D, tried one time. She completely read the recipe incorrectly. Instead of putting one-half of a cup of Schnapps in it, she put in two *whole* cups in it! I was just a kid, but I knew it was not right because I was getting drunk from the smell. She made a shit ton, so she gave some away. It became so popular that people wanted to buy it. My mom's mom, Grandma Marshall, came by at least once a week, picking up two or three more. Needless to say, we saw a lot of Grandma. We got really good Christmas presents from her that year. I loved Grandma, but she was batshit crazy. She got breast cancer and had to have a mastectomy. She named her "fake boobies" Willie Nelson, because she wanted him close to her heart. People say that she had no filter between her brain and mouth. Whatever the hell came out of her mouth was completely what she thought. Some people say that is where I got my attitude and loss of filter. I loved that woman.

She always was a joker in life. It hasn't stopped since her passing. Her favorite necklace came up missing from my sister's jewelry cabinet. It ended up buried in one of her plants. Heh heh on Debby. Then, however, our smoke alarms started going off in the middle of the night for no reason. Thanks, Grandma! These stories just make me think about her and all of my family. It makes me realize that Christmas is about thinking about your family, those who are here or who have passed. Just think of the good times. Even if there are bad memories, which we all have, leave them out of your head and heart. This is a good time to let bygones be bygones.

Just suck it up, my eggnog-filled buttercup. Put on your ugly sweater, and go to your stupid office parties and cookie exchanges. Hint: Don't mix eggnog with any real liquor. Eww! Just trust me on that one.

I just went to the Hancock family's Christmas party. Always fun and interesting. Always very loud. Good thing I had my allies in place to keep me from being overstimulated. The plan that Beth and I came up with really worked. I identified what was overstimulating, realized how it made me feel, and then made a plan for it. The dinner was in an old-school cafeteria with cinder-block walls. Every sound was amplified. There were thirty-five to forty adults and twenty kids. It was crowded and loud. I know that everyone was just catching up and having fun. I started to realize that I was getting overstimulated. My head started hurting, my stomach was in knots, and I couldn't get my thoughts straight. So I followed my plan and decided how to cope. I turned to my sister-in-law, Sarah, and started talking to her. Crisis avoided. The kids were playing games. It ended, and they got their prizes. One young boy got a recorder as a prize. He played it nonstop. I had enough and turned to Momma J and said, "If he doesn't stop, I'm going to jam that so far down his throat that he will shit it out later." Would I hurt anyone? No! I'm not capable of hurting anyone, especially a kid. Hey, I'm still learning how to cope.

It really made me think about how this situation, or one like it, will affect me in "real life." I have to be able to focus with distractions on the job and on the road. I get so frustrated because before I got sick with my liver, I could work twelve-hour days, go home, and clean house. I guess that is how I ended up sick—all stress, no rest.

Do I regret working so hard? Yes and no. I love working, but now I just have my book, a blog, and my disability check. Well, shit! I did it again. Letting my negative attitude bleed out. I like to blame it on my health, but that is bullshit. I've always been hard on myself. I would beat myself up over a B in school. I would try to argue it up to an A. I did it in work and to my employees. I need to apologize. Then I find myself torn. If that work reflects on me, then it should meet my standard.

I need to focus these feelings into things I love—my family, dogs, therapy, and cooking. Yes, Meghan, Shannon, and Beth, I did say that I love therapy. Just realize that you cannot hold that against me. Maybe I won't show this to you until it is finished. I don't want any of you getting a big head.

My family is my rock. They have seen me with tubes in my neck, stomach, and arms and with pressure splints on my legs. Everyone asks me how that makes me feel. It makes me feel sad—sad that the family I love so much had to see me like that. I, thankfully, cannot remember those times, but I have seen pictures of me shortly after coming through it. Don't get me wrong; friends visited me, too. For this, I am grateful as well. I am a blessed woman. You know, I talk about how I'm trying to be patient, but I never talk about how saintly my friends and family have to be. Still.

Let's lighten up. Momma J got me an electric pressure cooker for an early Christmas gift. I'm a chef, right, and a damn good one, too. Have I ever used a pressure cooker? Nope. The only memory of a pressure cooker was my five-foot-three mother standing over one with a fork on the "bobber" thing. "How did it turn out, Amanda?" you ask. Well, she didn't wait long enough, and the bobber flew across the room, as did the contents of the pot. You think she swears? Heh.

So it took me, Dan, Debby, and Janice to make this work. I read the directions. Dan read the directions. I called Debby. Dan ended up calling Janice to figure out how the damn thing works. We ended up having a great Italian beef sandwich with tater tots. Yes, I am a chef, but sometimes one just needs comfort food. Just this morning I had one of my favorite breakfast sandwiches: peanut butter and bananas. My sister used to make it for me and even cut the crust off of it. The only problem is that with every sandwich, she would take the first bite out of it. She said, "Amanda, I just want to make sure it's not poisoned." I was so naïve that I never thought, "Dipshit, she made the sandwich; it can't be poisoned." I never got the first drink of my beverage or the tip of the pie or cake. Sisterly love.

It is five days until Christmas, and I think I'm finally done. I was on a mission to make everything this year, which I have been able to accomplish. Beef jerky, cookies, peanut butter balls, dip mixes in ornaments, Bacon Jam, cocoa mixes, and chocolate dipped spoons. I also made some fruitcake, which may be a bit too strong. Oops. I had to soak the dried fruit in rum overnight. The cake was dense but called for another ¼ cup of rum. Whewee!

My grandmother was a hoot. She was strong and spoke her mind. Everyone says that she is where I lost my filter. Whatever shit came to her head came out of her mouth. Sound familiar? There is a story that there was one day when my grandpa came up and told her, "Get up off of your fat ass, and cook me some dinner." She was sitting on the porch in a lawn chair and stood up and took the chair, folded it up. and knocked him off the porch, breaking his ribs. "Who are you calling fat now?" My Grandma Marshall was amazing. She helped me get through my parents' divorce, always full of helpful advice. She had breast cancer and had to have a double mastectomy. She named her prosthetics Willie Nelson because she always wanted him close to her heart. She passed away on September 11, 2001. She had been in a coma for three weeks and had been in great amounts of pain. She passed just after the second plane hit the second tower. I told everyone that she was wanting to get to heaven to greet everyone with a joke and a hug. That day was difficult for the entire country, especially our family. We had to laugh because at her funeral she wanted the song, "There's Nothing I Can Do about It Now." Typical Grandma Marshall. Nope, but I bet there was a little old lady in heaven laughing her ass off at us.

Fourteen

Do I Think about Death?

Of course I think about death! I've almost died at least three times. Did I see a bright light? Nope. Did dead relatives talk to me? Yes, of course; it was Grandma Marshall. What did she say? "This is the third time you have almost died. Stop it! Go back, and take care of your family." Yeah, I haven't told anyone that. I had some seizures during my coma. My body was tired, and I was tired. People assume that people in comas are completely out of it. No! We can hear and think. The tests were showing that I had little brain function. Maybe at that point, it was depleted. When it came back, I was well aware of my surroundings. The doctor told Dan to bring in a radio because music stimulates brain activity. I have a killer song list, so I was loving it. Most people think that someone in a coma can't hear. Bullshit! I could "hear" what people were saying. Well, I could hear them mumble.

Now that I think about it, after I was trapped in a body that could not move, breathe on its own, or speak, it's no wonder why my first words were "No" and "Get the fuck out." I was finally free to open my eyes and talk. I even kicked out my doctor, who is one of the nicest people you'll ever meet. Everyone had questions and wanted to know what it's like to be in a coma. What kind of question is that? It is dark and scary! That is what a coma is. That is why I want that in this book. Comas are scary. You may not be conscious, but you are still a person, not a shell. I'm one of the fortunate ones who came out of the coma. Many people aren't that lucky. I don't think "lucky" is the right word; "fortunate" is. I would never wish that on someone.

I have learned a ton from the experience, mostly about my inner strength. I thought that before this, I was a pushover, but now I know how strong a will I have. I think I thought my kindness was weakness, much like people think crying shows weakness. It does not. Being kind is necessary for a good life. I think weakness is just a state of mind. There are people out there who have egos and think they are stronger because they are physically strong or may be wealthy. This thinking will end up backfiring in the end.

Strength is in your character and in your spirit, not in your pocketbook or muscles. Please understand that I am not objectifying anyone's experiences. I am just talking about what is on the inside. You might not have a penny to your name, but you will never see someone be taken advantage of. That is your confidence and strength coming out. Everyone has a passion for something, whether it be animals, civil rights, or people who are less fortunate.

Am I saying that there aren't bad people? Not at all. There are people everywhere who are trying to take advantage of others. Put on your strong-person pants, and stand up. Stop feeling sorry for yourself! Go show the world what you've got. Show them how strong you are. Especially here in the winter months, it is easy to be down in the dumps. You've spent all of your money on Christmas gifts, or you feel bad because you didn't have the money to buy gifts. Join the club. This time of year is bad for everyone at some point. It is cold and dreary. People just want to shut themselves in and feel sorry for themselves. It's true; our bodies do not like the cold. We ache, and our feelings are on the rocks. It's time to buck up and stretch. Put on something warm, and leave your house.

I have done a lot of crafts to help my mood. Do what I'm doing right now. Write down your feelings and thoughts. Start a journal or a blog, or both. I would say, "Write a book," but I don't need competition yet. Heh. Just do something that you like. I really suggest you help someone—anyone. It will help his or her inner strength, and yours as well. Go give someone confidence. Boost your own. Maybe the other person needs the same boost you do.

Fifteen

CHRISTMAS IS HERE AGAIN

Three days to go! Yes, I said three. Are you done with your shopping? Me neither. My credit is so bad that I have to use cash for everything. I spent my youth buying sunglasses, designer jeans, purses, and trips. I didn't know anything about a credit score. Well, now I know. When Dan and I were talking about getting married, he told me he needed my credit report. I was confused and insulted. At that point, I didn't realize that he would take on my debt when we got married. Oops.

Once I understood, I was on board. If you only carry cash, once it's gone, it's gone. Wise words by a very good lawyer that I happened to marry. After twelve years, I still carry cash. I do have a bank account, which I keep some spending money in. It is debit *only*! Smart advice, everyone.

Well, with Christmas comes another birthday. My birthday falls on January 6. Yes, I will be thirty-seven this year. What stinks is that every year: (1) I get older; and (2) I get the combined Christmas/ birthday gift. I get gypped. Yes, that is a word in my dictionary. It means "fucked over." Everyone gets two gifts, but I get just one. However, I do get two birthdays just a few days apart. My transplant was on January 11, so my liver is nineteen years old now. I'm sure my donor's family still misses him each year, but I hope they rest assured because he saved at least five lives. I'm not only thankful but also proud of him for being a donor. My family, especially Dan, missed me for nearly three years with my sickness. I was just a shell of a person for all of that time. Now I'm more of a person than they remembered. Heh. Lucky them.

This upcoming year is going to bring good things. I have been working with all of my therapists on making a new plan for my treatment. We are discussing aquatherapy once a week. Then, maybe I'll take off a couple of months so I can learn in "the real world." I think it is time. It is my goal to get a part-time job and start driving again. They have given me a lot of homework so that I can try things on my own. It should make me happy, but it makes me nervous.

Why? I'm not too sure. I have been so dependent on everyone, especially Dan, that the idea of standing up on my own is scary. It confuses me because I used to be so independent, but now I feel alone if not surrounded by people. Am I scared, or just nervous? I really don't know. Once again, I feel that I'm in that spot where I can see the light, but I cannot get to it. Then where do I end up? Sitting here at my computer, either writing this book or a blog. It's cathartic. Oh, yeah; I can use big words, too. In my heart I know that I'm ready to fly, but my head says otherwise. I've always been an overachiever to a fault. Speaking about caregivers, let's give them a chapter.

Sixteen

TAKE CARE OF THOSE WHO TAKE CARE OF US

I should not be writing this chapter; this is Dan's wheelhouse. This is a difficult topic for me. It was hard for me to watch the toll that my illness took on him. I can't imagine how he felt, watching me struggle. It was hard for me to struggle, but he still has the burden of driving me around, paying all the bills, and trying to work on top of that.

While I was sick, a group of my high-school friends put on a fundraiser to help raise money for my medical bills. Of course, I had no idea because I was so sick. There were three friends whom Dan had never met who got in touch and asked his permission. They did a spaghetti dinner and raised a ton of money.

I consider them caregivers. They were not hands-on, per se, but they took it on themselves to help me out. I am so humbled because I hadn't talked to many of them in years. I have been trying to personally thank them lately. One of my best friends, Hayley, has been there since grade school. Hayley and my friend Angie led the fundraiser. Anna (fo fanna) began as an employee and ended up being another best friend.

I cannot express how important it is to thank everyone. Just a text is not enough; call friends, and thank them in person. There are websites where you can nominate a caregiver to be recognized in public or even to win meals or prizes.

Seventeen

Happy New Year

Well, here we are: 2017. Here's hoping it's better than the last three have been for me. I have already listed my goals, but I feel like I need to review them daily. You should, too. I've decided to put mine in my phone so I have it all the time. To be completely honest, I just had to look them back up so that I could put them in my phone without being a liar. I think maybe I need to add that to my list. I don't have a habit of lying. In fact, I've never been a liar. I tried a few times as a kid and realized I was terrible at it.

So I am getting older in four days. Today is January second. My birthday is on the sixth, and what I call my second birthday is on the eleventh. Why two birthdays? The first is my "birth day," and the second is the day I got my liver transplant. I like to celebrate both. In fact, I would not be alive right now if it hadn't been for my liver donor. He was seventeen, so now my liver is nineteen. That makes my body thirty-seven. Yuck! I have trouble with that fact. I just remember making fun of both my husband and my sister when they turned forty. Now I am the one creeping up on it. If I average it, I'm only twenty-eight. So I'm going to say that I have the body of a twenty-eight-year-old. That is true enough, right? Just nod your head: "Yes, Amanda." Thank you for feeding my illusion.

It is now 2017, and I started this book in June of 2016. That means I have been working on this book for seven months. I have been told by my therapists that I can read it, but I cannot edit it. Apparently, it shows my progress in my thought process. I know that it has changed a ton. I can see it in my therapy progress notes. In fact, they are wanting me to maybe take a few months off so I can try out my skills in the "real world." That makes me nervous and scared. Mostly nervous. Why? This year my goals are to drive and get a job again. Frankly, this scares the shit out of me. I haven't driven a car in three years. The last job I had was owning a restaurant. How am I going to handle this?

It confuses me because three years ago, I would work twelve hours a day, drive home, clean up, make something to eat, shower, and get up and do it again. Dan and other family and friends tend to remind me how that is how I ended up so sick. Yep, they are right. Do I like to admit that? Nope. I do, however, know that is the case.

Dan let me drive just a block, and I panicked the whole time. I didn't let him know, but just the idea that I could hit something makes me a nervous wreck. My depth perception has not developed quite as fast as I would like. I still have difficulty with my reaction time. Stopping is still a hardship for me. This timing is hard for me to figure out. This is why I am doing time trials in my occupational and SLP therapies. SLP stands for speech language pathology. Beth times me on different tasks. With her I also have to multitask between different trials, including math, categories, and word forming out of limited letters. That is my favorite task. Shannon, my occupational therapist, times me on my fine motor skills. This includes things such as putting pegs into holes, fastening clothespins on different posts, and throwing blocks over a board to see how many I can get in a certain amount of time. I know it sounds goofy, but doing these tasks while being timed is quite taxing. She and I also work on my arm flexibility, eye/hand coordination, and grip strength. I have a physical therapist also, Meghan (the Boss), who helps with my core strength, balance, and overall endurance. All these ladies are doing their damnedest to get me ready for the tasks I'm about to have to encounter when I am out of therapy. Soon I will be starting aquatherapy and counseling, both of which I feel will help with my anxiety and overall nervousness about being on my own. I also feel concerned because I have been so dependent, and now, I am supposed to figure it out. I know I am not going to be left hanging out there, but I haven't been independent for three years now. Scary shit! I'm constantly telling people, "Suck it up, buttercup." Now, I guess I have to do it. Ever want to kick your own ass? Yep, me too—right now. Do as I say, not as I do, right? That's like saying, "Because I said so!" Yeah, Mom, that's for you.

Now that I think about it, I hope you get this far into this book. I know I said in the beginning I didn't have the cognition that I do now. Everyone who has read it so far has said that it seems like it has been written by three different people. Now, I feel like they are saying that I have multiple personalities—not really, but maybe that's why they suggested counseling. Hmm…

I always wonder how everyone's life is going. That is why I blog, too. I love writing, but this does not give me the feedback that the blog does. If someone does not like what I say, they can post right back at me. Good, yes. Bad, yes. It can either be an ego boost or a blow. There are often words of encouragement, usually. I've never had unhappy readers, but it could be that they are just being nice. I am guessing that my readers are like me and don't get their panties in a wad. Yes, I know that's so nineties, but I am a nineties baby. I was born on January 6, 1980, so I don't really remember the eighties. That is why I align myself with the nineties kids. Yes—grunge music, *The*

Fresh Prince of Bel-Air, The Wonder Years, Seinfeld, and *Twin Peaks.* I bet you haven't thought of about those things in in sixteen years. How about Cabbage Patch Kids?

So I will start aquatherapy next Tuesday. I need to get the dreaded swimsuit. Ugh. I have never looked good in a swimsuit. Never, even when I weighed 145 pounds. Big thighs, no boobs, and no butt. Now, I have too much of it all. For God's sake, it is 45° F out there, and the stores are already putting out swimsuits. I've noticed that people still have their Christmas decorations out. Off on a tangent. This is something I am supposed to be looking out for when I begin to edit this book. I do not think I should change the way it is written, because I feel like it shows my progress. Once you read it, you can let me know. I tend to let my mind wander. You have probably noticed this by now.

Well, now that I've gotten off track, let's talk food. Yes, again. I am not supposed to do that. Oops! I got new toys for Christmas. I know that I was just complaining about Christmas stuff. Well, this is my book, so…blah. Momma J and Dad #2 (Janice and Frank) got me an electric pressure cooker. It took me, Dan, Debby, and finally Janice to work the damn thing. Even though Dan and I had read the directions several times, we couldn't get it to work. So I called my sister (the all-knowing), and she didn't know, either. We had to swallow our pride and call Janice. She told us what we were doing wrong, and voilà, it was perfect. Have I used it since? Nope. They are coming over today, so maybe I can get a hands-on lesson.

I did an interview with the paper yesterday with my culinary professor and good friend. We made my stir-fry recipe, which is a few chapters back. Then, we made a cheesecake that I came up with. It is a Brie/cream cheese cake with sautéed apples and pomegranate reduction. I made the crust out of pecans, walnuts, honey, cream, and bread flour. It is kind of a cheesecake on top of a big cookie. I'm terrible with interviews, so I am anxious to see how it turns out.

Eighteen

A Cheesecake That Deserves Its Own Chapter

So I just described this cheesecake; now you get the story, and maybe the recipe. The base is actually Dan's recipe. It is the typical four-ingredient base with a butter/graham cracker crust. I decided to take that base and kick it up a notch. I lost my palate while being sick, so now that I can taste, I take every opportunity to make everything I touch have a little extra kick to it. I decided that the cream cheese could use some help, so I added Brie to it. I couldn't do the usual crust, so I decided to add a cookie texture to it. That is where the nuts, honey, cream, and bread flour come in. It makes, quite literally, a cookie. To add extra flavor, I sautéed apples and added a pomegranate glaze to the top. Then, this time, Dan was nice enough to smoke it over orange wood, apples and all.

Before I get into it, I want to explain how I lost my palate. I was having trouble eating because my liver disease had advanced so far that I stopped eating. After my transplant I went into a coma. All of my feedings were coming through a nasogastric tube. I had to get a tracheotomy, so then my nutrition was coming in through a feeding tube in my stomach. Long story short, I didn't eat for several months. Once I got my trach out, I could only have cold broth. It took me a lot of therapy to be able to eat again. That is why this book is so food-oriented.

So, let's talk cheesecake. Bear with me; the recipe is long.

The Best Cheesecake You Will Ever Make!
Hands Down

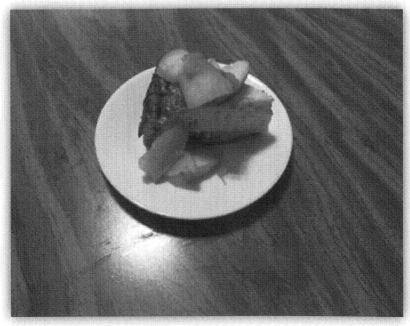

smoked Brie cheesecake with smoked apples and a balsamic reduction

This recipe is long, so get over it; you will be proud of the ending. Trust me! This recipe needs a seven-inch springform pan. You will do this in several steps that need to be followed.

Preheat your oven to 325° F. You will start with the crust, filling, and then the topping.

<u>Crust</u>
Ingredients:

- 1 cup butter
- ¾ cup sugar
- ½ cup heavy cream
- 2 oz. each of pecans and walnuts

Directions:

- Grind nuts in food processor; place in a bowl.
- Add flour and sugar into the bowl.
- Stir in melted butter, honey, and cream.
- Press into a greased springform.
- Blind bake, which means to bake it once without opening the oven, for 15 minutes.
- Let cool while making the filling.

Filling ingredients:

- 1 cup butter, softened
- 3 eggs
- 2 8-oz. blocks cream cheese
- 1 8-oz. round Brie
- ¾ cup sugar or local honey
- ½ cup cream
- ½ tsp. almond or vanilla extract

Directions:
- Cream softened butter, cream cheese, and Brie.
- Add eggs, one at a time.

- Add cream and sugar.
- Add vanilla extract.
- Mix until well incorporated, and put into the cooled shell.
- Bake for 1 hour at 325° F.

Topping ingredients:

- 3 sliced Granny Smith apples
- Lemon for keeping the apples from turning brown
- Butter for coating the skillet
- 2 Tbsps. sugar
- Cinnamon, fresh nutmeg, apple pie spice, and so forth
- Melt the butter in the skillet. Add the apples and lemon juice. Add the sugar and cinnamon. Sauté until soft but not mushy.

Balsamic topping:

- Add 1 Tbsp. butter to a nonstick skillet.
- Let brown, and then add balsamic vinegar. I use pomegranate vinegar.

Final assembly:

- Let the cheesecake cool completely. Warm up the apples. Top the cheesecake with the apples. Top with the vinegar.

Hopefully, this has inspired you to make this cheesecake. To kick it up a notch, Dan and I smoked our cheesecake over orange wood. We smoked the apples separately. Once put together, it made the most amazing flavor profile of a cheesecake that I have ever encountered, if I do say so myself.

Nineteen

The First Birthday Has Come and Passed

So, Amanda, how does it feel to be thirty-seven? I am sore and grumpy. Everyone says age is just a state of mind. Bullshit! It is cold and dreary.

I did, however, get some great gifts. My mom got me a French coffee press. I have never had one, so I'm very excited. Debby got me a new stand mixer. Mine bit the dust. I wore it out in the store and at home. My mom has never made pasta, so I think we will do that soon. My sister delivered Mom here as a birthday gift, too. She is always a pleasure to have here. Debby said she is staying for six weeks. Um, no. I ran it across Dan, and he said, "Um...I don't think so." My sister wants us to dry her some pasta. I tried one time, to no avail. I decided to hang it in the guest closet. That went south, literally. Most of it fell off onto the floor. Oops! Now that Mom is here, that is not an option. Maybe the best way to dry it would be to nest it. Hmm. That might just be the next chapter.

With my next birthday, I want to celebrate organ donation. It just came out that in France, there is an opt-out option. This means that people are considered organ donors until they opt out. In every state in America, a person has to opt in by putting it on his or her driver's license.

I was lucky enough to be the first on the list for a donor. I have not had contact with the family of my donor because it is too close to the time of my transplant and his death. The only way to contact the donor family is to write a letter to the family and send it through the Indiana Donor Network. If the family members want to have contact, they can choose to write back. No one knows who the donor is, not even the nurses. The only people who do know are the transplant doctors and the harvest staff. I have mixed emotions about meeting the family. I have a friend whose mother had a liver transplant and decided she wanted to meet the family. It has only been two years, but I still get emotional thinking about his lost life and how he saved mine. I still struggle with guilt. I know that I shouldn't, but I can't help it. This young gentleman single-handedly saved five lives. I hope that his family knows his contribution to so many lives. I am forever grateful. I am dedicated to supporting the donation program for life. I guess my life is living proof. There is no guessing—I *am* proof. I hope you, as a reader, can see this. By the request (more like demand) of my therapists, I cannot edit the content of the book until I have a copy of the original in full. How long will the book be? When does it end? I guess it will end when I feel like I have completed all of my goals for the book. I am hoping that I will be able to work and drive soon. Then I will feel more complete. I am scared and nervous about the "real world." Scared, but more nervous. Why? Because it has been three years since I have driven or worked. I used to work for twelve hours running the restaurant; then, I drove home and would cook and clean. Eight hours later, I would do it again. Maybe that is why I got so sick. I know that I have already talked about this, but just keep in mind that you need to take care of yourself. Don't get caught up in life, or it will take over your life.

Twenty

How to Make Pasta

Yes, you will be able to make your own by the end of this chapter. My birthday gifts! Momma D is here, and we are going to make pasta tomorrow! My good friend Aimee Blume sent me her recipe for perfect pasta. I am going to pass this wealth on to you. You are welcome.

Aimee Blume's Pasta Recipe
The easiest pasta you can make!
This recipe is a bit different because the ingredients are relative to each other. Bear with me.

Ingredients:

- 1 cup all-purpose flour
- 1 egg
- 1 Tbsp. olive oil
- Mix the ingredients in a mixer with a hook until well mixed.

- Sprinkle salt and water to make a stiff dough.
- Remove from the bowl. Wrap in plastic wrap, and let rest (at room temperature) for at least 30 minutes.
- By hand, roll out the dough thin enough to go through a pasta roller. Once it is thin enough, roll it through a clean pasta roller until it is at the desired thickness.
- If cooking soon, drop the pasta into a pot of boiling, salted water.
- Be sure that whatever dish you choose to make is very close to being finished before dropping your pasta.
- Your pasta will cook in just a few minutes.
- I would suggest a very light sauce because the pasta is fragile—maybe an oil, lemon, and herb sauce.

When drying:

- Separate the strands and hang in a clean, cool, dry place.
- Also, the pasta can be nested by wrapping it around a can and letting it sit—again, in a clean, cool, dry place.
- Always store your pasta in an airtight container to ensure it stays fresh.
- Cook your dried pasta just a little longer than your fresh because it is still a fresh product. Always use well-salted water. Do *not* use oil in your water.

A person can always tell when the pasta is fresh. It has a different bite and texture. Only cook your pasta al dente, which means "to the tooth." I will make a promise to you that you will never want store-bought pasta again. Once you get good at it, you can fill your pasta with the ricotta cheese that you learned to make in earlier chapters.

If you make your pasta wide enough, you can make fresh lasagna. Just imagine: fresh pasta and fresh cheese—and you made it all!

Today, January 11, 2017, is a big day for me. Not only am I celebrating my second anniversary with my new liver, but I am also making pasta with my mom. To make it special, we are using duck eggs from my sister's farm. Momma D is so proud because she feeds those ducks every day and collects their eggs whenever they lay. She and I haven't rolled them yet, so I will let you know how it goes.

Twenty One

It Is Time for New Experiences

You know me by now, always saying it is time to try new things. I decided to do the same thing. I will be a hypocrite if I don't do it. What did I do? I started going to a counselor and started aqua-therapy. Both ended up being painful. I had no clue that I would be emotional after counseling, but I was. This time is always hard for me. The weather is dreary and cold. My bones and muscles hurt and ache. I have noticed that everyone around me is feeling this way. Still battling with guilt and grief, I know that this is my time to put my head up and start to be proud of myself. I have problems doing that in good conscience. I know it sounds counterproductive, but I have always had a guilt complex.

I then thought I could take this out in the pool. Pools are fun, right? Yes…and no. The first steps into the pool revealed that the temperature of the water was 90° F and like the perfect bath. Then, I realized that I float. I am no longer the lean brick of muscle I was in my twenties. Nope. I am fifty pounds heavier. I keep telling myself that it's all muscle. Bullshit, Amanda. My mom worked with a lady who, every Christmas, gained ten pounds of "muscle." Heh heh.

My therapist was very nice and asked me if I could swim. Rolling my eyes, I said, "Of course." Two steps in, my fat ass was slip-sliding around that pool. She kept telling me that the pool was not slick; my balance was just that bad. Great. Boss tells me I don't have good balance on the ground, and now, Chris, my aquatic therapist, says I don't have balance in the water? How the hell do I get around? Then, I got to thinking that I haven't swum since high school. Now, I spend my time on a floaty with a drink in the cupholder. I am too lazy to get out to get my next drink. I just keep a cooler that I can put on the side and paddle to. No wonder there is no muscle there.

Tonight I start back to AceCare. That is the volunteer physical therapy class that I do once a week. I am curious as to how I will feel after doing aquatic therapy just a few days ago. I'm still sore, especially my arms. While in the water, I knew my legs would get sore, but I did not think about my arms. I didn't realize that I was using my arms to keep my balance. So, I guess tonight, I need to work on balance.

Since I have started my aquatic therapy, I have not been participating in my outpatient program. This is due to the fact that Medicare limits the number of visits per month; we have to split visits between therapy on land and in the water. I thought it was no big deal. I was wrong. Obviously, I have worse balance in the water than on the land. I guess we will see. I will let you know in the next chapter.

I am still waiting on my vocational rehabilitation assessment results. I have received my basic result, but not the final draft. It will finally give me the timeline for my driving evaluation and my job evaluation as well. I was told that my job goals were going to be difficult to accomplish because my goal is to teach people with disabilities how to cook. I am aware that this is a lofty goal, but you know me by now. I cannot do anything the easy way. It is really not lofty, but it seems like it from a provider standpoint.

I was a "provider," meaning that I had responsibility for those who were deemed by the state to need twenty-four-hour care. When certified by the state, the providing company must follow state-mandated regulations to function. These providers are frequently audited by an inspector to ensure compliance.

Why am I explaining this? To be able to complete this task, my "providers," being vocational rehabilitation providers, must meet their regulations to ensure that my plan is complete and beneficial to me. They have to make sure that I am strong and can endure the work environment. As I have stated in the past, I have a deficiency in my level of endurance. I tire easily. As you know by now, I have some problems with staying on task without overstimulation. It is not that I cannot stay on task, but I can be overstimulated by constant loud noises. It was never a problem until my brain injury.

My brain functions as quickly, but emotionally, I get frustrated, causing me to get nervous and shaky, with headaches and nausea. There are times when this can throw me off my task. My speech therapist and I have come up with a plan. I have to define what is causing my overstimulation, define how I feel, and determine what I can do to cope. I know this can only help if I know what I am up against. Yes and no. If I know, I can have allies to talk to. If I don't know, I can find a place to cool down or remove myself from the situation. I understand that this is not always feasible, so I can just take a break for a few minutes.

As far as driving goes, I need to have another eye exam. I also need to practice my reaction timing. I don't trust myself on the road yet. It would be detrimental for me to put myself in the position to get hurt or hurt someone else. My therapists have given me tests to help with my timing. Most include reading. Being in physical therapy also challenges my depth perception when I walk backward and turn my head back and forth while walking. I also have to sidestep while keeping a safe distance from the wall. Walking in the pool has proven to test my spatial issues just by dealing with the motion of the water. It is in a stainless-steel pool. It looks, and is, clean. It is, however, slick as shit. How do I know? I grew up on a farm…lots of shit around farms. Guess what? You step in it, too. It is slick, too.

Enough about shit. Let's talk about what it means to have spatial issues. I had an eye doctor explain to me that if you are looking at a 3-D picture, and you see nothing, your eyes isn't working altogether. He went on to say that if you move the picture, your brain will "pick up" the signal, and you will see the picture. I know that is not the way it works, but it is the best way that I can describe it. It has to do with the way your brain transmits spatial items to your brain. I lost most of my spatial awareness during my brain injury. I have trouble knowing how close things are, especially monochromatic items.

During my occupational therapy sessions, I have to stand in front of a wall full of holes for pegs. I must reach as high as I can with my left arm and place the pegs in the holes. Why my left arm? This is the arm that is affected by my ODS the most. The pegs challenge my vision. It is very hard to keep my balance and know how close I am to the board. This is part of the reason I cannot drive. I get it, but I am very frustrated. I feel like that is understandable.

To help, Momma D is visiting and reteaching me how to knit and crochet. I used to do a lot of knitting, especially in dialysis. After my transplant I did not have the motivation or desire to do it. As I'm not doing therapy every week, Momma D and I sat down, and she started helping me get reacclimated to holding the knitting needles and crochet hook. I had no clue how much dexterity I have lost. Just from the fifteen minutes we did, I got frustrated and am sore.

I feel like this has become my "bitch and complain" chapter. I am grateful for my progress; however, I need to find an outlet. I do blog, which helps. Maybe keeping notes will help me with my counseling. I sent my counselor a copy of this book. He finds me interesting. Should that worry me? I guess that is his job. He doesn't seem like the kind of guy to bullshit me. He was a counselor in a halfway house for bad guys. Like, really bad guys. I asked him how it compared to the children's group homes, just because I wondered if it caused the same amount of stress.

Twenty Two

LEARNING HOW TO KNIT AND CROCHET

I think we will be learning together on this one. While I was in dialysis, I learned how to knit. Both my mom and sister knit. I thought it would be perfect for me to learn, too. Back then, while I was very sick, I still had my dexterity. Dialysis goes on for three to four hours at a time. This gave me time to get really good at the skill. My mom originally taught me, and then my friend Anna helped me hone my skills.

I'm always amazed at how Anna knits. She is superfast and supertalented. I was amazed at how she was working on a cowl at a rate that I cannot explain. I am so jealous of her skills. She has been knitting for twelve years. Ever since my injury, I have trouble with my hand-eye coordination.

I know I have to get a lot of practice. Holding the needles in each hand has proven to be more difficult than I had imagined. Learning how to knit means learning a whole new language. If patterns were written outright, they would be forever long. There are abbreviations for each stitch, like K (for knit). There are abbreviations for everything. It is like learning an entire new way of thinking. I compare it to learning how to read music. Different notes mean different tones. The same is much like knitting, such as "K2 P1" means "knit two, and then purl one." Can I describe this to you? Nope. This is why Momma D bought me *Knitting for Beginners*, published by Future. I could not find an author, but it seems to be a collaboration of several master knitters. They all seem like masters to teach me how to knit again. Once again I find myself getting frustrated and confused by this process. The frustration comes from the fact that I used to be so coordinated. It made me feel whole. My intelligence feels compromised, too. I have never been one to have difficulty learning. Now it feels like everything takes twice as long to sink in. I understand that it is part of my "disability." I'm starting to feel like I use that as an excuse.

All of this time, I have been an advocate for keeping your head up and working to get stronger. I feel like I have let myself down. I certainly hope that I have not let you, the reader, down as well.

With the help of my friends, I am trying to find a place to do cooking classes. I have been asked by several people to do cooking classes. This is my dream. I sincerely want to teach people with disabilities how to cook. I know, I know, I used the "D" word again, but I do not know how else to say it. As a social worker, I worked with people with all types of disabilities, especially autism. I also understand the undertaking of such a large goal. I am ready for it. I know that I will need caregiver help and a facility that can be used for such tasks. I am sure there will be insurance issues as well. So much to think about. So much planning.

In therapy, I am given tasks to organize, at which I happen to be really good. All things need to be alphabetically organized or in numerical order. Sometimes I do this to a fault. It can be distracting, which I am also working to cope with. So many problems. At this point I am motivated to accomplish everything; however, it is easy to feel beaten down. This, to me, feels like the hardest part of my recovery thus far—knowing in my head that I have the ability but not quite being able to tap into it. This makes me wonder if everyone feels like this. When I think back to my younger years, I was constantly beating myself up for not being better. Even when I was at the top of my class, I felt like I had fallen short. I think this is the shit I need to talk to my counselor about. Hopefully I remember to take notes.

I have strayed from the title of this chapter, but sometimes I realize that learning how to knit is as boring as reading about it. Granted, I am still going to learn; I just needed to work through my head the reasons that I am so hard on myself. I realize I talk about therapy a ton, but it is all that I have known for months now—an entire year now. I just realized, while writing my blog, that I keep trying to get into the "real world." Holy shit, I *am* in the real world. I cook, clean, and take out the trash. The only skills I am lacking are a job and driving skills. Hopefully I will find a job and some driving lessons soon. I have been asked to conduct some cooking classes. I just can't find a venue at which to teach.

As you are well aware, teaching is my goal. Teaching and writing have become my main goals. I received a French press for Christmas. Now I am constantly jacked up with caffeine—lucky you. I am supposed to be working on attention span. Coffee probably isn't a good mix. Neither is Red Bull. Oops!

Twenty Three

Today Is Inauguration Day

It is a gloomy day for Hillary and Bernie supporters. Yeah, yeah, it's Trump. I do not like politics and typically refuse to talk or write about them, but today is the day. It doesn't help that the weather is dark and gloomy. The best aspect of this ceremony is "The Notorious RBG." Who is that? Only the smartest, most cunning woman to ever serve on our Supreme Court. Ruth Bader Ginsberg makes me smile. She is a strong, small woman who is one of the smartest women I have ever studied. I said that she makes me smile; that is because she wears a doily around her neck over her robe. It just reassures me that smart women can be respected, no matter what their appearance. I hope people see me that way.

On another note, today is National Cheese Day! All I can think of is dill Havarti, Swiss, cheddar, Brie, bleu...the list is endless. Now, I just need some crackers and wine. I think that it is amazing that just mentioning food can make a person crave certain things. It is the same with smells.

It has been a few days since I have written. Plenty has happened. Most of January is gone. Thus far, it has been eventful for us here in the Hancock clan. Well, I mean for me.

I know that I have listed all of my goals. Guess what? I am one step closer to my goals. I spent most of the past two weeks making phone calls to potential job coach providers. Also, I have an appointment with the driver's education division of Easter Seals. This a great facility that provides services to people with disabilities. I actually worked there for several years. It did not end well, but I completely appreciate the services they provide to the Evansville community.

I have been given the names of three job services with which I will interview to find the best fit. I used to interview people all the time. Now, it is different because it directly affects my future in the job world. Admittedly, I am nervous. I don't know why; I just am. The idea of being back in the workforce scares the shit out of me. The last job I had, I was the owner of an Italian restaurant and deli. Not only was I my own boss, but I had a crew of ten employees under me. This being said, I'm not sure how to take direction from a boss. The only boss I have is "the Boss" in my physical therapy. The only reason I call her the Boss is because she makes me work to reach my goals. She says that is her job, but I know better than that.

It is the same with Shannon ("Sit up straight, sister") and "Concentrate" Beth. Without them and my AceCare family, I couldn't have come as far as I have. I don't think that I have talked much about AceCare. This is a program run by physical therapy students who are essentially doing "practice." It is their job to help us complete different tasks to gain strength, endurance, or balance, depending on each of our needs.

There are six of us, all with different diagnoses. Most have experienced strokes. Some have Parkinson's disease. I am the only one with a brain injury. Many people consider me to be a TBI (traumatic brain injury) patient, but mine was acquired from my liver transplant. That is my ODS.

Most people still do not understand ODS, and there is really no easy way to explain it. Even many medical professionals do not know about it or understand it. There are few people who contract it and live. In 2015 four liver transplants done at the University of Indiana ended up getting ODS. Some professionals prefer to call it central pontine myelinolysis. That, to me, sounds even more confusing.

The best way to explain it is to imagine an electrical wire. These wires are always coated in rubber to keep the electricity contained. Our brains act the same way—coated. When the coating gets disrupted, the wires cross. It happens in the pons portion of the brain, which is right at the brain stem.

What does this have to do with Inauguration Day? Not a damn thing. Once again, I got distracted by something more important. I should say, "Something I feel is more important." It is my book, you know.

Everyone keeps asking me when I am going to finish this book. I'm not sure. The title is *The Best Is Yet to Come*. But how am I supposed to know when the best is here? I think it is getting closer. Why? I have interviewed two potential job placement providers, and I have found one that I really like. On to the next chapter in my life.

Twenty Four

THING ARE CHANGING FASTER THAN I IMAGINED

So far, I have interviewed two potential job placement providers. Like I said, there is one lady whom I really liked. I feel like she is one of the few people who understand my goal in my "real world" life. She and I spoke at great length about my desire to teach people with disabilities how to cook. As we spoke, we came up with a plan to possibly *create* a job for me to do. There is not currently a market for this type of plan because no one has ever thought of it in this area. Typically, this area is traditional in its thoughts about what a disability looks like. I get dirty looks for parking in the "handicapped" spots. I know that people look at me and think, *She's not disabled.* And no, I do not look "disabled," but I still have difficulty walking long distances. When I don't need the space, I choose not to use it.

At any rate, I have learned to not pay attention to it anymore. This morning I found a quote by the great Nelson Mandela. He said, "The more informed you are, the less arrogant and aggressive you are." I could only hope that everyone could follow that mantra.

I also found another quote that really spoke to my heart. "Help people even when you know they can't help you back." That quote really spoke to my social-work side. I spent nine years in group homes and individuals' homes who needed help. Social work is often a thankless job; however, I now know that is not why I chose to do that line of work. I feel like I needed them maybe even more than they needed me!

The second job counselor did not impress me much; however, she did give me insight into the fact that I can make money while still drawing my disability. I have spoken to my vocational rehabilitation counselor, and she says that is a real possibility. I feel like things are starting to come around for me.

Another good thing happening for me is that I have been approved to take a driving evaluation. This not only makes me happy, but it also makes me scared and mostly nervous. When I first got my license, I was sixteen and invincible. Now, I have too much to live for. Come on—I survived a liver transplant with complications. I am writing a book and a daily blog. I'm getting my ducks in a row for possible job opportunities.

So how is this affecting me emotionally? I am trying to take it one step at a time and remember where I've been and where I am planning on going. It is a shame that I can't remember most of the past two years. My long-term memory is great, but my short-term memory is still sketchy. I have been told that it is better that I do not remember. In the beginning the doctors were afraid that I would end up with PTSD if I started remembering everything.

There are parts of me that say that I remember, but I've been told that is part of the whole deal. The only things that I remember are hearing songs while in my coma. I know, I know, people say that is not possible, but it is. Do I remember all the songs? Nope. But I remember the vibration of the music. It was very close to my bed, so I could feel it. Most people do not realize how much that affected me. But it did.

Today, February 2, 2017, marks the two-year anniversary of me opening my eyes from the coma. Talk about being heavy on my heart. That affected me more than I thought it would. I don't remember much, but everyone says that is a good thing. Just over the last two years, my short-term memory is coming back. I do remember being delirious at RHI and thinking it was 2008. It took me several months to figure out it was already 2015. I was convinced that they had me in the basement when there was no basement. It got worse, I think, when I went to the nursing facility closer to home. I had a problem learning where exactly where I was, even though I was close to home. This is where I really started working on my walking skills with a man who would put five-pound weights on my ankles and make me walk. By the time I left, I was a walking miracle.

An even harder transition was coming home. I remembered the place, but I had trouble navigating it. I know it sounds funny, but I legitimately could not find my way around. I had trouble realizing that I was home. It had been eight months since I had seen the inside of my home. I thought my guest bedroom was my room. I forgot what it was like to sleep on a real bed.

I'm still amazed at how much I changed in that period of time. I had to have in-home care for the first few months because I was too weak to go to real therapy. I was still having to use a wheelchair for trips to the grocery store. There was one time when I got cocky and fell in the parking lot. Luckily, Dan is a strong man and was able to pick me up and get me back into the truck. We learned our lesson. From that point on, we had the chair with us.

Even when I first started AceCare, the free physical therapy class I go to weekly, I was going in a wheelchair. They did a video of the class, and there was Dan, faithfully following me with my chair. I had to

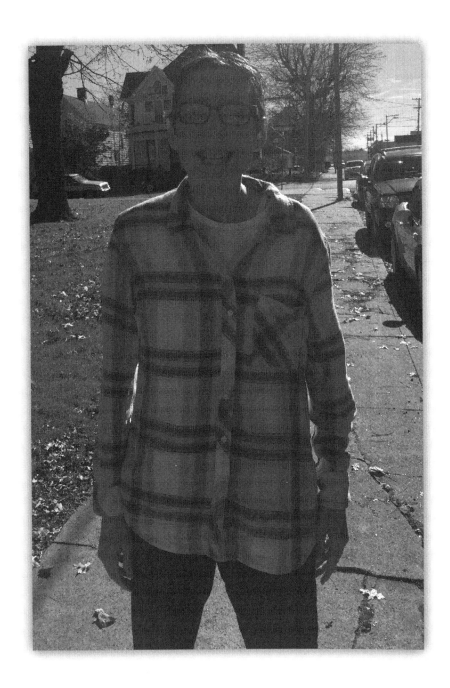

depend on it daily. They gradually started working with me without the chair. That was a *huge* step for me! The ability to walk on my own was amazing. Of course, they had a gait belt on me to make sure that someone could catch me if I toppled over. Gradually I started surpassing the other folks in the class. Everyone gives me a hard time, because they say that I'm making the class harder for everyone. It has gotten to the point where they have a program just for me. Last week I was walking with three-pound ankle weights and had someone behind me with a resistance band pulling on me. Talk about hard! Everyone in the group has become very close friends. We all do the same program, but we are at different levels. At first, they had me doing wall push-ups. That became too easy, so we went out to the conference area, and they had me do push-ups on the back of the chair. As if that wasn't hard enough, I had to do it with one foot up behind me. That proved to be too hard, so I was able to just put one foot on its tiptoe.

Needless to say, I was sore as shit the next day! I plan on continuing with AceCare, but as far as my other therapies go…well, I think they feel like I'm graduating from them. This is exciting, but it makes me realize that I am becoming more independent. I think that I will continue with aquatic therapy and my counseling. Other doors are opening up for me everywhere. I'm meeting with a lady tomorrow who has offered me the opportunity to teach people with disabilities how to cook. This class will be held on Tuesday of this upcoming week. Then on Wednesday, I will be meeting with another possible provider to work on my cooking classes. They only do cold dishes, so that will be yet another challenge.

I've gotten to the point where I welcome challenges. My driving evaluation comes on Monday of next week. Talk about challenges. I am not sure if this is a physical challenge or a mental one. I tend to psych myself over things that I really want to accomplish. I know that if I need to get lessons, they will provide them to me. In my head, I feel like I should be able to do it the first go-around. I have to remind myself that it has been three years since I have driven. That doesn't mean I can't do it; it just means I have to be careful.

This afternoon I met with the nice lady who has organized the cooking class that I am doing later this week. I am both excited and nervous. I'm happy that I will be working with people with financial difficulties and also with disabilities. These people live in a community that has connected apartments because at some point, they have been homeless.

The following Tuesday, about a week after setting up the class, we went to the facility. I will admit, at the beginning, I was very nervous. When Dan and I walked in, the ladies were talking about a recent stabbing in that neighborhood. I automatically was taken out of my shoes when I heard that. One of the ladies actually had a child involved in the event. Apparently her daughter was the person who came across it and ended up saving the life of the victim. Needless to say, I was ready to leave.

After getting to know these women, I was inspired to keep on doing this. Each lady wanted to participate and wanted to help cook. Many had not ever eaten zucchini. This was exciting to me because I love to introduce people to new things. They made a lasagna, which was raffled off to one of the new participants. At the end everyone had good questions and asked me to come back. This made me very happy, of course.

On this Wednesday, I will be meeting with another potential facility where I may have an opportunity to cook as well. It has gotten to the point where I have a calendar in three different places. One goes on my refrigerator, one on my phone, and one I carry with me all the time. It almost feels like I am working full time again. Between therapies, potential job interviews, and my driving lessons, I am a busy lady.

Well, my meeting went very well. It is not the same type of facility as the last class that I taught. This is more of a meeting place for underprivileged people. This facility has a common area, a food bank, weekly potlucks, and weekly Narcotics Anonymous meetings. To teach here I would have to commit to doing it for free. It will be up to me to find participants. I feel like I have enough contacts to do that. I understand that to do this, I will have to budget so I will not become a charity case myself. My other option is to spend money to buy liability insurance, just in case someone gets hurt or sick from the food. I will also have to get what is called a ServSafe Food Handler Certificate. This will make sure with the state that I, indeed, am safe with food. I think everyone serving food should have to have this certification.

I am very proud of how far I have come so far. Just think—two years ago I was still in a wheelchair. I'm painfully reminded every morning while getting dressed; all of my clothes still have my name stickers on the backs of each of them.

I am gradually graduating from my therapies. Meghan, my physical therapist; Shannon, my occupational therapist; and Beth, my SLP, are not discharging me, but they are giving me home exercise programs (HEPs) to do at home while working on getting a job and driving evaluation. Each discipline has a different set for me to do. So, in essence, I'm not discharged, just temporarily graduated. I still plan on doing my aquatic therapy and my weekly AceCare sessions.

This will still keep me busy and active; however, like I said, I've become a very busy lady. The ladies in my regular therapies will continue to reevaluate me every so often. The way that Medicare is set up, I have to show monthly progress to keep my benefits.

How exciting! Even if it is only $1,000 a month, that is no joke, as I haven't made any money in three years. Obviously I can only work two to three hours a day, as I haven't built up my endurance as much as I should. The Boss has given me enough homework to keep me in shape for a while.

Along with that, I will be working on my speech and occupational therapy homework, too. It is my goal to actually write out a set workout regimen for each day. I figure if I can endure four days of workouts plus AceCare, I will be building strength and endurance every week. I guess that means that I will have to set up a goal to organize all of that, too. So much for a weekend off. That is just fine by me. I love a challenge, maybe to a fault.

I also guess that I need to work on my résumé. Last time I looked at it was four years ago. As I was running a restaurant, I never thought I would need a résumé. I had it in my head that I would never have to work for someone again. Um, well, I guess plans can change at the drop of a hat. That's the story of my life.

Twenty Five

Even More Changes Are Coming!

I *finally* took my driving evaluation just yesterday. It is already February 14, which is both Valentine's Day and National Organ Donor Day! I never care too much about Valentine's Day. I kind of feel like it is just a holiday for the greeting-card stores. National Organ Donor Day is a different story. As important as it is to remember those of us fortunate enough to receive a donation, it is probably more important to recognize the donors and/or their families. It is easy to just assume that someone had to die to donate, but that is not the case. Many times a portion of a liver can be donated, or even a kidney.

Many people still do not know that donation is an option. In many European countries, everyone is considered a donor unless he or she requests otherwise. Obviously, in my opinion, that is the only option that makes sense. However, I am one of the fortunate people to be on the receiving end of a donation.

Back to my driving evaluation. My instructor said that I did very well, but I still needed three to five hours of driving lessons for more practice. I, of course, was disappointed, but I understand how important it is that I not hurt myself or anyone else.

Once again, I'm nervous because next Monday I have to go for my FCE. An FCE is a functional capacity evaluation. This is a series of exercises to make sure that I can complete everything needed for a potential work situation. This makes me miss the Boss telling me to work harder. I feel like I need to call her for some encouragement. Knowing her, she will just say, "Suck it up, buttercup!"

I'm a little worried because I just posted about her in my blog, and I am going to see her tonight at AceCare. Oops. I did buy a bunch of Girl Scout cookies from her kid, so maybe she will go easy on me this go-around.

So, I haven't written in a week or so. Not because I did not want to, but my ass has been superbusy. I had my FCE. How did it go? I have no fucking idea. The gentleman was very nice, but because of the testing, he could not give me any results. The only thing he could say to me was that I was "more than sedentary." How am I supposed to know what that means? He was able to tell me that I could lift forty pounds from floor to waist, thirty pounds overhead, twenty-five pounds carrying a box one hundred feet, and finally pushing and pulling a fifty-pound sled twenty-five feet back and forth three times.

I have never been so sore in my life. The following day I had a doctor appointment, a counseling appointment, and aquatic therapy. Talk about needing a rest. Nope. Yesterday, Wednesday, I did three loads of laundry and two loads of dishes. Dan and I did fit in some time to go on a small date. We went and saw *The Lego Batman Movie*. Cheesy for adults, but good, mindless fun.

Today is Thursday, February, 23, 2017. I will be going to one of my favorite things: AceCare. It is another way for us to get more exercise. It is a great free program for people who may not qualify for outpatient therapies. I'm lucky enough to be able to benefit from it all.

Also, I have chosen a job coach with Goodwill. She and I are pretty close in age and have very similar likes. She is very supportive of my goal to want to teach people with disabilities how to cook. Hell, at this point, I just want to teach anyone how to enjoy their food more.

And I did my driving evaluation and have been approved for three to five hours of lessons. At that point, I should be able to drive on my own. It is a lot for me to handle in such a short time. That is why I am very happy to have a good therapist. Yes, I even have a head therapist. I feel like to be completely healed, it must be without and within. I need to cross-stitch that on a pillowcase.

I have recently run across photos and videos of myself while in the very beginning of my recovery. I even have my first recorded steps. I even have the first time I could lift my head and grasp a hairbrush. I know they all seem like baby steps, but that is exactly what they are.

I am proud of the steps that I have made, but I also understand that I could not have done it without the amazing team of family, friends, and professionals who surround me. I know that I piss and moan about how hard they are on me, but I wouldn't have it any other way.

I take a few days off writing, and a ton of things happen. After AceCare last night I have changed my monthly goals. Last night we had an actual yoga class. Oh, my goodness, I had so much fun. On the television it looks so easy; however, in reality. it leaves you sore as shit. I have never had the ability to meditate; however, Mac, the instructor made it easy. I'm not one to have the ability to clear my mind. As we sat there, I was able to start to clear my head and focus on the people around me, my caregivers, and myself.

That is something I haven't taken time to do. I've spent so much time trying to recover that I have forgotten to really think about how I feel inside my brain. It seems like everything has been focused on healing my body. I've completely forgotten about my spiritual and mental well-being.

On another positive note, I have made several appointments for myself this upcoming month. I am officially meeting with my new job coach, Brandy, twice over the next two weeks. I've also received a phone call from my driving instructor, Rusty. Also, starting next week, I will be doing my driving lessons. The only assessment I will need to do is a "benefit evaluation." This will let me know how much I can earn without affecting my benefits.

I've decided to continue with my therapies, including occupational therapy, SLP, physical therapy, AceCare, and aquatic therapy. I have been learning how to schedule my own time, which has always been a difficult task for me. Beth, my speech therapist, and I have been working on this for several months. Now, it is time for me to show her that I can do it on my own. I have a cooking class forming. It is just a matter of finding the facility to do it. I have spoken to a foundation that is eager to invite my crew in. I have convinced my physical therapists at AceCare that they need me to teach them how to cook. Most of them are college students on limited budgets. This gives me a great challenge, not only for my time management but also for my budgeting skills.

Even though my favorite genre to cook is Asian, especially Thai, they all want me to cook Italian. It is only because I once owned an Italian market and deli; they think I'm an Italian food guru. This adds extra pressure because they expect more from me for just that reason.

I do have a class set up, and they want me to make Stromboli with them. Most local restaurants just put meat, cheese, and sauce on a bun and toast it. I use all of those things, but I bake them in a homemade pizza dough.

I've recently reconnected with a supersweet nurse who took care of me while I was in the TICU in Indy. I never knew her, but she knew me well. She told me the last time she saw me, I could not speak. Now, I speak too much—sometimes even putting my foot in my mouth or up my ass. It has been really nice actually getting to know her. She is now a nurse in Pennsylvania, where she is from.

I lastly have been talking to my sister, Debby, about our ancestry. She got her DNA tested and learned a bit more about our family. Her test said that we are 67 percent from Great Britain; 16 percent from France; 9 percent from the Italy/Greece area; 2 percent Scandinavian; 2 percent Irish; 1 percent Spanish; and less than 1 percent from Poland/Ukraine, Finland, and the Caucuses. In my mind, that makes us quite the mix.

I think that makes my sister the supersmart one; me the big, stubborn one; Momma D the old country smart one; and poor Dan and John stuck in the middle of this mess. I haven't asked Dan how he feels about being stuck in the middle, but I can only imagine what he thinks about it. Poor John, Debby's husband, is so-laid back, I can only image he sits back and soaks it in. I don't even want to think about what our in-laws think about us.

Twenty Six

I Think I'm Finally Getting Used to "Real Life"

As the days go by, I feel myself changing. So far, I have met my daily goal to blog, do yoga, and write in this book. Today, March 1, I went to take one of my driving lessons. I did so well, my instructor said that if I do as well tomorrow, he will sign me off as passing! I cannot tell you how excited I am to do this. I haven't driven on my own for over three years now.

Dan has to go to court as I am driving. I asked him if I could drive home. He is so tired of being my chauffeur, so he is ecstatic to finally have a driver. He has been driving me around since I started dialysis in 2014.

I have also met with my job coach, Brandy. I really like her. Not only are we close in age, but she is also as motivated for me to reach my goals as I am. Next week, on March 8, I will be meeting with local business owners and human resource managers. Am I nervous? Why, yes, I am. I know that there is no reason for me to be, because I have a ton of experience and an education to back me up. There is just something in my head holding me back.

Even as a kid, I was very hard on myself. If I got a B on my report card, I was disappointed. I was so undecided about college that I'm afraid my parents gave up on me. Now that I reread this, I realize that I am more than that. Dan just found my diploma from Murray State University, in Murray, Kentucky. Of course, I get the jokes that it's not valid because I got it in Kentucky. Well, it is just as good as yours. It doesn't say that I was on the dean's list every semester that I was there. By the way, Dan was born in the great Commonwealth of Kentucky. That is where we got married as well. We did have to swear that we were not relatives.

I think that I am finally getting to the point where I feel fulfilled. For so long I felt like only half of a person because of the situation I was in. I just keep telling everyone, "I just got dealt a bad hand. It is my responsibility to make it a better hand." I feel like all the shit I've had to crawl through is part of my redemption. I do not expect anyone to understand this; it is pretty obscure thinking. With the support of Dan and my family, I chose to fight. The last thing I said to Dan before I went into a coma was, "If something happens to me, you just let me fight." I meant that when I said it. I had no idea of the pain that would cause him, but he did exactly what I told him to do.

Now, there are times when I feel terrible, as if I had put too much pressure on him. In my mind, I was trying to make it easier. Who knew that I would be stubborn enough to fight through eight months in a hospital setting and three years of intense therapy? I knew it. I can't tell you how, but I knew that I am made for more than the terrible hand I was dealt. I think everyone should think more like this. Mostly, people get stuck in a rut, feeling sorry for themselves and doing nothing about it.

I feel like I'm proof of that. Just in the past two weeks, I have taken three driving lessons and regained the ability to drive on my own. I cannot begin to tell you how much of a relief that is to me. Dan has had to drive me around for at least three years while I have been sick. Now, it is my turn to drive him around!

Admittedly, it has been a while since I have written. This means that I haven't kept up with my goals to write every day. There is a good reason for that. Not only have I regained my ability to drive, I have also taken steps toward getting a job. Last Wednesday, I met with between ten and fifteen human-resource people and local business owners. I had two minutes to present myself, my résumé, my experience, and my vision for employment to this committee. I *nailed* it! Everyone was interested and had several questions for me. I was able to answer each question. They also provided me with possible leads for employers and contacts of people whom I could call. The following day I met with my job coach, Brandy, and we were able to look up possible outlets for potential employment.

I have been persistent in my goal to teach people with disabilities how to cook. Thus far, I have taught one class, but it was for people who were, or have been, homeless at some point. It was a very successful class in that each person there wanted to participate and chip in to the final project. It was a hit. The ladies made a Crock-Pot lasagna with my instruction. It turned out great, as they ate every bit of it. The group is currently trying to find a date to invite me back.

As I have been talking to other professionals about my goal to teach, many providers of services for people with disabilities have shown interest in wanting to take my classes as well. Together we decided it could be beneficial for them to learn a few easy dishes that they could teach their clients as well. Running with this idea, I have booked a class with the college students who teach my physical therapy classes through the University of Evansville. They have caught wind of the fact that I used to own my own Italian restaurant, so they think that is my specialty.

Though I am good at it, Italian cooking is not my favorite. At any rate, they want me to teach them how to make Stromboli. The typical Stromboli in this area is a sandwich of beef/sausage mix, cheese, pepperoni, and sauce in a bun. The way I make mine is that I take all these ingredients and bake them wrapped inside homemade pizza dough. To finish it off, I brush the outside with a garlic/olive oil mixture. It makes for a very flavorful and appealing look and taste. This is a group of college students who work with folks like me, who just need a little help getting stronger. A few of the single students have stated that "when" they get girlfriends or boyfriends, they want to be able to make at least one thing with which they could impress potential significant others. It makes me laugh, and I tell them that is how I landed Dan.

I will never tell them that when we met, I could not cook at all. I had to let my sister teach me how to cook. Shh…I will never admit to that to her face. She will not know until she reads this book. As well as the students in AceCare, where I get my physical therapy, many of the participants have shown interest in taking a cooking class with me.

Now that I have my license, I'm a driving machine. Dan's grandfather passed away, and his funeral was yesterday. Dan asked me to drive, and I was happy to. It was an hour and a half drive to Earlington, Kentucky. Where is that? I cannot even begin to tell you. I just followed Dan's directions and the signs.

Speaking of being a driving machine, this weekend, I'm trying to convince Dan to let me drive back to my hometown. West Frankfort, Illinois, is a small town in Southern Illinois. It is an old coal mine town. As the mines began to close, the town began to fail. It is in the middle of cornfields and meth labs. I know that sounds harsh, but it unfortunately is the truth.

My immediate family still lives there. Momma D, Debby, John, and Emily have a nice home in the country. Well, I say that, but most of West Frankfort is country land. Mostly, since the coal miners left, it has become a land of corn and soybeans. A few of my friends still live there but have jobs in the surrounding small cities. There is Carbondale, where the University of Southern Illinois is. Then, there is Marion, which houses a minor league baseball team.

I briefly went to SIU but realized it was too close to home, and I couldn't find a good job around there.

I ended up moving to Evansville to chase a job. I had started my social-work degree at Murray State University but did not have the financing to finish it. That is when I started an entry-level job with an agency that helped people with physical and mental disabilities in their homes. After I met Dan, I felt like I needed to finish my degree because I got tired of telling people that I was married to a lawyer and I hadn't finished college yet. After rearranging my work schedule, I was able to take both online and TV-based classes in an extension facility in Henderson, Kentucky.

This allowed me to climb the ranks within the social-work world. It is a very fulfilling profession but has a high burnout rate. I lasted seven and a half years and then had to bail. That is what brought me to culinary school. I neglected to mention that I met Dan here, too. Online, in fact. This was back when it wasn't cool to meet online. In fact, I posted a profile as a bet. I had a friend convince me that I could just do it to find out where people hung out around here. I had only been here a few times and didn't know where to go.

When Dan and I were both matched on Yahoo, neither of us cared for each other. He thought I was too tall and young. I thought he was too short and old, and he had bright red hair. Somehow, we both kept getting matched up. Finally, he convinced me to give him my number. As soon as I did, my phone rang. I guess now that I think about it, he must have been excited to meet me. I didn't tell him that I had already scheduled a date with someone else that night. I just told him that I might need to cancel because my sister might come in.

Long story short, he showed up in ragged, patched jeans and ate off my plate. Not impressive, right? Well, he asked me if I had ever played blackjack. I had not. We went to a boat, and he gave me forty dollars and taught me how to play. Once I got the hang of it, I ended up winning $150 back. I think that's when he decided he wanted to marry me. After six months and after his attempts to show his cooking skills, he asked me to marry him.

The proposal site was beautiful. It was at a riverside park looking over the new Owensboro bridge. It was perfect…that is, until I ruined his proposal. As soon as I figured out what was going on, I got both nervous and excited. The second I saw the ring, I ripped it out of his hand, jammed it on my finger, and started jumping up and down. Then, I screamed, as loud as I could, "Yes!" I think I startled Dan, because he just looked at me and said, "So, um…OK, will you marry me?" I think I maybe had gone a little over the top at that point. After being together for thirteen years and married for twelve, I think we will make it.

Twenty Seven

I Think the Best Is Coming Faster Than I Expected!

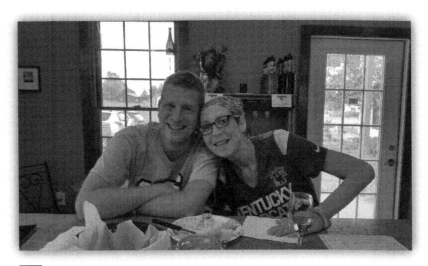

Today is March 29, 2017. It's been roughly eight months from the beginning of my venture to write this book. I have to take breaks here and there because I have created a busy life for myself! Since the last time I have written, I have gotten my license, a car, liability insurance, an LLC, and a job offer. I have taught two cooking classes and have been offered the opportunity for a place to continuing to cook as long as I want.

Patchwork is a location that helps a population that is underserved. I recently taught a class of college students whom wanted to learn how to make my Vecchio's Stromboli. I was lucky enough to have two of my best friends and fellow chefs join me to teach the class. Aimee Blume was my culinary professor, and she also writes for our local paper. Chef Jessica Keys is a chef who graduated from Sullivan University in Louisville, Kentucky. She was also my right hand while I owned Vecchio's.

To me, they had three of the best chefs in the area teaching them baking, knife skills, and the proper way to dress a salad. I think that we were all amazed that many of the students had no clue what a garlic chive was or even what asparagus was or what it tastes like. I had no clue what that feeling was. It made me so proud of all of them!

Chef Jess (I'm just going to call her Jess from here on out) has made as many Stromboli as I have while working for and with me. She took the lead on teaching them how to roll out dough, what "gluten" is, and why it is important to baking. While this was going on, Chef Aimee (just Aimee from here on) spent this time cooking the meat, and I began heating up the sauce. Dan and I opened the pepperoni and provolone cheese.

Once this was all done, the students could assemble their creations. Dan and I washed, chopped, and assembled the salad. Aimee and I created a salad dressing from a high-end Italian olive oil, pomegranate balsamic vinegar, salt, Greek seasoning, and the garlic chives. Before Aimee chopped the chives, I took them around for the students to smell and taste. Once Dan was finished chopping the asparagus that he had grilled that morning, we let them try what they were like grilled. As I said, many had never tasted the vegetable before this point.

We had made enough food that we were able to donate the leftovers to the facility. As Dan and I had taken donations from our pantry, many of the students did as well. As professional chefs we have two goals: (1) Make food look good and taste even better than it looks; and (2) not only cook the food, but also teach people the importance of fresh food, nutrition, and taste, compared to the usual processed foods of today.

"Suck it up, buttercup!" That is what I usually tell everyone else, but lately, I have to tell myself that! It's April 9, 2017. I think I have been writing this book for a year now. Just in the past two months, I have gotten my driver's license back, received a car, gotten a job, taught two cooking classes, and have booked at least three more.

Just next week I have a meeting with my job coach, a trial run for the cooking class I'm teaching later in the week, a date to entertain my Momma D, and appointments to teach a class, get a haircut and color, and then observe/help my boss with a class that she is teaching! I fought and prayed for this day. Now, I cannot say that I regret it, but I sure am tired. I am honored that the local bakery has asked me to start making my focaccia bread for its sandwiches.

Everyone is telling me that I am spreading myself out too thin. I like to deny it, but I'm starting to think they might be right. How confusing! Just when I think that I've found the best, I start to wonder if this is it. Dan and I were able to go for a day out. No dogs, no phones, just us!

We went to French Lick and West Baden. These are two of our favorite places to go. This is an area in Southern Indiana that has just started coming back to life. These were two famous hotels in the days of Al Capone. They were built on hot springs, which became popular in those times for cleansing the body. Even though it has become popular, it feels like it belongs to only us. We eat at our favorite restaurants and sit under the famous West Baden Dome!

I have been talking to a publisher for this book, but I don't know what is a good deal and what is not. I feel like it is coming time to close this chapter. Dan has moved his office and is getting more and more business. I have a car, a job, and the potential to become a "real culinary teacher." I am closer to my friends and family more than ever. I still call my dog Lulu or Lucifer. I have a nice house, and my Momma D is coming to visit.

Back when I started this book and this journey, I had just come home from being in a hospital setting for eight months. These were just ideas that I was jotting down on paper because I didn't have the dexterity to be able to type. Look at me now! I have been places recently where people have not recognized me.

I guess I am just saying that this is bittersweet. I have put my whole life on these pages. What now? Has the best really come?

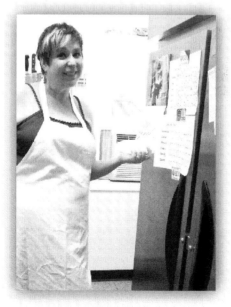

Made in the USA
Middletown, DE
21 November 2017